MW00862330

ADVANCED
FETAL MONITORING COURSE

Student Materials

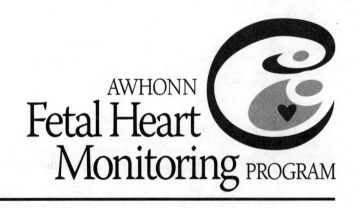

AWHONN
Fetal Heart Monitoring PROGRAM

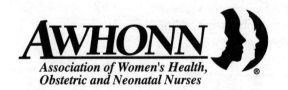

AWHONN
Association of Women's Health,
Obstetric and Neonatal Nurses

KENDALL/HUNT PUBLISHING COMPANY
4050 Westmark Drive   Dubuque, Iowa 52002

CONTENTS

Target Audience

The Advanced Fetal Monitoring Course (AFMC) is based on educational theory. The instructional design incorporates critical thinking and decision making and is specifically designed for clinicians with previous fetal heart monitoring (FHM) experience. Residents, physicians, LPNs and LVNs may also take the course. Prior completion of the Intermediate Fetal Monitoring Course is *not* a requirement for Advanced Fetal Monitoring Course attendance; however, AWHONN strongly recommends completion of a basic fetal monitoring course prior to attendance. To facilitate successful completion of the course, participants are expected, prior to attending the course to review *Fetal Heart Monitoring Principles and Practices, Current Edition,* and the AFMC study guide and outline, which include suggested readings. Although the content of the workshop is comprehensive, specific patient care responsibilities vary according to institution, state, province or region. Participants of the course are advised to be familiar with institutional responsibilities, as well as competence criteria and measurement.

Acknowledgement of Commercial Support

This CE/CME activity has been created without commercial support.

Sponsorship Statement

The CE activity is co-sponsored by the Association of Women's Health, Obstetric and Neonatal Nurses (AWHONN) and by the Professional Education Services Group (PESG).

Learning Objectives

At the conclusion of this continuing medical education activity, participants should be able to:

- Identify basic physiologic principles underlying fetal heart monitoring.
- Describe advanced physiologic principles of maternal and fetal oxygen transfer and acid-base balance.
- Describe advanced concepts in antenatal testing, including analysis and interpretation of biophysical profiles and complex antenatal fetal heart monitoring tracings.
- Identify physiologic principles, goals and interventions for patients undergoing antenatal testing.
- Evaluate the effectiveness of interventions for patients undergoing antenatal testing.
- Compare and contrast physiologic principles and causes of adult cardiac dysrhythmias with fetal cardiac dysrhythmias.
- Analyze fetal cardiac dysrhythmias patterns and describe outcomes associated with these patterns.
- Analyze complex fetal heart monitoring patterns, including uterine rupture, maternal-fetal hemorrhage, and abruption, utilizing National Institute of Child Health and Development (NICHD) FHM nomenclature/definitions.
- Apply perinatal risk management principles, communication techniques and documentation strategies related to complex and challenging patient care scenarios.

Content Validation Statement

It is the policy of AWHONN and PESG to review and certify that the content contained in this CE/CME activity is based on sound, scientific, evidence-based medicine. All recommendations involving clinical medicine in this CE/CME activity are based on evidence that is accepted within the profession of medicine as adequate justification for their indications and contraindications in the care of patients.

AWHONN and PESG further assert that all scientific research referred to, reported, or used in this CE/CME activity in support or justification of a patient care recommendation conforms to the generally accepted standards of experimental design, data collection, and analysis. Moreover, AWHONN and PESG establishes that the content contained herein conforms to the Definition of CE as defined by the American Nurses Credentialing Center (ANCC) and the Definition of CME as defined by the Accreditation Council for Continuing Medical Education (ACCME).

Disclosure Statement

It is the policy of Professional Education Services Group that the faculty and sponsor disclose real or apparent conflicts of interest relating to the topics of this educational activity and also disclose discussions of unlabeled/unapproved uses of drugs or devices during their presentations. Detailed disclosures will be made available during the live program.

Conflict-of-Interest Resolution Statement

When individuals in a position to control content have reported financial relationships with one or more commercial interests, as listed in their particular disclosure, AWHONN and PESG will work with them to resolve such conflicts to ensure that the content presented is free from commercial bias. The content of this presentation was vetted by the following mechanisms and modified as required to meet this standard:

- Content peer review by external topic expert
- Content validation by external topic expert and internal AWHONN and PESG clinical staff

Educational Peer Review Disclosure PESG reports the following:

- **William Mencia, MD,**
  Vice President of Medical Affairs/CME Director
  Dr. Mencia has no significant financial relationships to disclose.
- **Lawrence Devoe, MD**
  Dr. Devoe has no significant financial relationships to disclose.

Accreditation Information

AWHONN is accredited as a provider of continuing education (CE) in nursing by the American Nurses Credentialing Center's Commission on Accreditation. AWHONN also holds California, Alabama and Florida BRN numbers: California CE provider #CEP580, Alabama #ABNP0058, and Florida BON# 50-4759.

The maximum CE credit that can be earned while attending the Intermediate Fetal Monitoring Course is 18.3 AWHONN contact hours.

Professional Education Services Group is accredited by the Accreditation Council for Continuing Medical Education (ACCME) to provide continuing medical education for physicians. This activity has been planned and implemented in accordance with the Essential Areas and policies of the ACCME.

Credit Designation Statement

Physicians: Professional Education Services Group designates this educational activity for a maximum of 15.25 category 1 credits toward the AMA Physician's Recognition Award. Each physician should claim only those credits that he/she actually spent in the activity.

DISCLAIMER

This course and all accompanying materials (publication) were developed by AWHONN, the Association of Women's Health, Obstetric and Neonatal Nurses, as an educational resource for fetal heart monitoring. It presents general methods and techniques of practice that are currently acceptable, based on current research and used by recognized authorities. Proper care of individual patients may depend on many individual factors to be considered in clinical practice, as well as professional judgment in the techniques described herein. Clinical circumstances naturally vary, and professionals must use their own best judgment in accordance with the patients' needs and preferences, professional standards and institutional rules. Variations and innovations that are consistent with law, and that demonstrably improve the quality of patient care, should be encouraged.

AWHONN has sought to confirm the accuracy of the information presented herein and to describe generally accepted practices. However, neither AWHONN nor PESG are responsible for errors or omissions or for any consequences from application of the information in this resource and makes no warranty, expressed or implied, with respect to the contents of the publication.

Competent clinical practice depends on a broad array of personal characteristics, training, judgment, professional skills and institutional processes. This publication is simply one of many information resources. This publication is not intended to replace ongoing evaluation of knowledge and skills in the clinical setting. Nor has it been designed for use in hiring, promotion or termination decisions or in resolving legal disputes or issues of liability.

AWHONN and PESG believe that drug selection and dosage set forth in this text are in accordance with current recommendations and practice at the time of publication. However, in view of ongoing research, changes in government regulations, and the constant flow of information relating to drug therapy and drug reactions, the reader is urged to check other information available in other published sources for each drug for potential changes in indications, dosages, and for added warnings, and precautions. This is particularly important when the recommended agent is a new or infrequently employed drug. In addition, appropriate medication use may depend on unique factors such as individuals' health status, other medication use, and other factors which the professional must consider in clinical practice.

RESOURCES AND REFERENCE MATERIALS

BASELINE VARIABILITY

The numbers (1) through (4) included in the following cells correspond to the numbers encircled on the Visual Assessment of Variability Scale.

Amplitude of FHR Change	Former AWHONN Baseline LTV Description	NICHD Baseline Variability Description
(1) Undetectable from baseline	Decreased/Minimal	Absent
(2) Visually detectable from baseline, ≤5 bpm	Decreased/Minimal	Minimal
(3) 6–25 bpm	Average/Within Normal Limits	Moderate
(4) >25 bpm	Marked/Saltatory	Marked

Source: Adapted from Electronic fetal heart monitoring: Research guidelines for interpretation, National Institutes of Child Health and Human Development Research Planning Workshop, 1997, *Journal of Obstetric, Gynecologic and Neonatal Nursing, 26*(6), 635–640. Copyright © AWHONN.

Note: The exact language in the 1997 NICHD paper regarding minimal variability is "greater than undetectable" and less than or equal to 5 bpm. AWHONN has chosen the equivalent term "visually detectable" to clearly differentiate the definition of minimal variability from the definition of "absent variability," avoid confusion for users new to the NICHD terminology, and emphasize the visual determination of variability.

VISUAL ASSESSMENT OF VARIABILITY SCALE

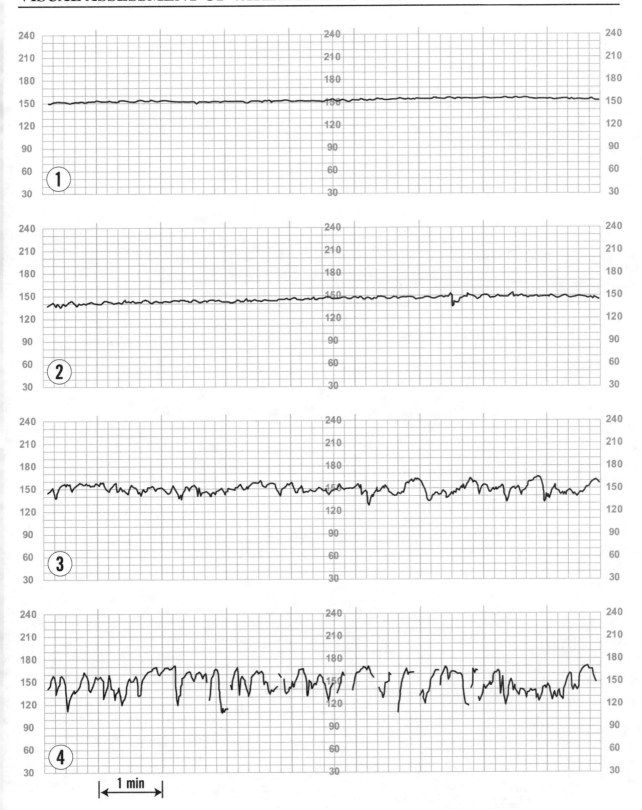

1 min

Source: Adapted from Electronic fetal heart monitoring: Research guidelines for interpretation, National Institutes of Child Health and Human Development Research Planning Workshop, 1997, Journal of Obstetric, Gynecologic and Neonatal Nursing, 26(6), 635–640. Copyright © AWHONN.

INTERPRETATION AND SUGGESTED MANAGEMENT
FOR BIOPHYSICAL PROFILE SCORES

Score	Interpretation	Management
10 / 10 8 / 10 (normal AFV) 8 / 8 (NST not done)	No acute or chronic asphyxia	No fetal indication exists for intervention. Conduct serial testing as indicated by condition.
8 / 10 (abnormal AFV)	No acute asphyxia; low risk of chronic hypoxia	Deliver if oligohydramnios present. Use serial testing if <36 weeks. Twice weekly for diabetics and patients ≥41 weeks gestation.
6 / 10 (normal AFV)	Chronic asphyxia suspected	Deliver if fetus is ≥36 weeks and favorable conditions. Repeat test in 4–6 hours if >36 weeks and L/S ratio <2.0.
4 / 10 (normal AFV)	Chronic asphyxia suspected	Deliver if fetus is >36 weeks. Repeat test same day if <32 weeks.
2 / 10	Chronic asphyxia suspected	Extend observation period to 120 minutes. Deliver if score is ≤4 regardless of gestational age.
0 / 10	Chronic asphyxia suspected	Deliver regardless of gestational age if persistent score ≤4.

AFV = amniotic fluid volume
NST = nonstress test
Source: Adapted from Manning, F. A., Platt, L. D., & Sipos, L. (1980). Antepartum fetal evaluation: Development of a biophysical profile. *American Journal of Obstetrics and Gynecology, 136,* 787–795.; Manning, F. A., Harmon, C. R., Morrison, I., et al., (1990). Fetal assessment based on biophysical profile scoring: IV. An analysis of perinatal morbidity and mortality. *American Journal of Obstetrics and Gynecology, 162,* 703–709.
© 2006 AWHONN. Reprinted from AWHONN's *Fetal Heart Monitoring Principles and Practices, Third Edition* (2003). Table 12-5, p. 275.

FETAL HEART RATE CHARACTERISTICS AND PATTERNS: NICHD (1997)

Term	Definition
Baseline Rate	Approximate mean FHR rounded to increments of 5 bpm during a 10-minute segment, excluding periodic or episodic changes, periods of marked variability, and segments of baseline that differs by >25 bpm. In any 10-minute window, the minimum baseline duration must be at least 2 minutes or the baseline for that period is indeterminate. In this case, one may need to refer to the previous 10-minute segment for determination of the baseline.
Bradycardia	Baseline rate of <110 bpm.
Tachycardia	Baseline rate of >160 bpm.
Baseline Variability	Fluctuations in the baseline FHR of 2 cycles per minute or greater. These fluctuations are irregular in amplitude and frequency and are visually quantified as the amplitude of the peak to trough in bpm.
- Absent variability	Amplitude range undetectable.
- Minimal variability	Amplitude range visually detectable (>undetectable) but ≤5 bpm.
- Moderate variability	Amplitude range 6–25 bpm.
- Marked variability	Amplitude range >25 bpm.
Acceleration	Visually apparent **abrupt** increase (onset to peak is <30 seconds) in FHR above baseline. The increase is calculated from the most recently determined portion of the baseline. Acme is ≥15 bpm. above the baseline and lasts ≥15 seconds and <2 minutes from the onset to return to baseline. Before 32 weeks of gestation, an acme ≥10 bpm above the baseline and duration of ≥10 seconds is an acceleration.
Prolonged acceleration	Acceleration ≥2 minutes and <10 minutes duration.
Early deceleration	Visually apparent **gradual** decrease (onset to nadir is ≥30 seconds) of the FHR and return to baseline associated with a uterine contraction. This decrease is calculated from the most recently determined portion of the baseline. It is coincident in timing, with the nadir of deceleration occurring at the same time as the peak of the contraction. In most cases, the onset, nadir, and recovery of the deceleration are coincident with the beginning, peak, and ending of the contraction, respectively.

(continued)

Late deceleration	Visually apparent *gradual* decrease (onset to nadir is ≥30 seconds) of the FHR and return to baseline associated with a uterine contraction. This decrease is calculated from the most recently determined portion of the baseline. It is delayed in timing, with the nadir of deceleration occurring after the peak of the contraction. In most cases, the onset, nadir, and recovery of the deceleration occur after the onset, peak, and ending of the contraction, respectively.
Variable deceleration	Visually apparent *abrupt* decrease (onset to beginning of nadir is <30 seconds) in FHR below baseline. The decrease is calculated from the most recently determined portion of the baseline. Decrease is ≥15 bpm, lasting ≥15 seconds and <2 minutes from onset to return to baseline. When variable decelerations are associated with uterine contractions, their onset, depth, and duration vary with successive uterine contractions.
Prolonged deceleration	Visually apparent decrease in FHR below baseline. The decrease is calculated from the most recently determined portion of the baseline. Decrease is ≥15 bpm, lasting ≥2 minutes but <10 minutes from onset to return to baseline.

Source: From the National Institute of Child Health and Human Development Research Planning Workshop: Electronic fetal heart rate monitoring: Research guidelines for interpretation. *American Journal of Obstetrics and Gynecology* (1997) 177(6), 1,385–1,390; and *Journal of Obstetric, Gynecologic and Neonatal Nursing* (1997), 26(6) 635–640.

REFERENCES

Adelsperger, D., & Waymire, V.J. (2003). Physiological interventions for fetal heart rate patterns. In N. Feinstein, K.L. Torgersen, & J. Atterbury (Eds.), *Fetal heart monitoring principles and practices* (3rd ed., pp. 159–175). Dubuque, IA: Kendall/Hunt.

American Academy of Pediatrics and American College of Obstetricians and Gynecologists (2002). *Guidelines for Perinatal Care* (5th ed). Washington, D. C.: Author.

American College of Obstetricians and Gynecologists (ACOG) (1999). *Antepartum fetal surveillance* (Practice Bulletin No. 9). Washington, D.C.: Author.

American College of Obstetricians and Gynecologists. (1995). *Fetal heart rate patterns: Monitoring, interpretation and management* (Technical Bulletin No. 207). Washington, D.C.: Author.

American College of Obstetricians and Gynecologists. (2001). *Fetal pulse oximetry* (Committee Opinion No. 258). Washington, D.C.: Author.

American College of Obstetricians and Gynecologists. (2003). *Neonatal encephalopathy and cerebral palsy: Defining the pathogenesis and pathophysiology.* Washington, D.C.: Author.

American College of Obstetricians and Gynecologists. (2005). *Screening tests for birth defects* (Patient Education Series). Washington, D.C.: Author.

American Heart Association & American Academy of Pediatrics. (2000). *Neonatal resuscitation textbook* (4th ed.). Washington. D.C.: Author.

American Nurses Association. (2004). *Nursing: Scope and standards of practice.* Washington, D.C.: Author.

Armour, K. (2004). Antepartum maternal–fetal assessment. *AWHONN Lifelines, 8,* 232–240.

Association of Women's Health, Obstetric, and Neonatal Nurses. (1998). *Clinical competencies and education guide: Limited ultrasound examinations in obstetric, gynecological/infertility settings.* Author: Washington, D.C.

Association of Women's Health, Obstetrics and Neonatal Nurses. (2003). *Standards for professional nursing practice in the care of women and newborns* (6th ed.). Washington, D.C.: Author.

Atterbury, J.L., Mikkelsen, G.M., & Santa-Donato, A. (2003). Antepartum fetal assessment. In N. Feinstein, K.L. Torgersen, & J.L. Atterbury (Eds.), *Fetal heart monitoring principles and practices* (3rd ed., pp. 261–288). Dubuque, Iowa: Kendall/Hunt.

AWHONN. (1997a). *Fetal heart monitoring: Principles and practices.* 2nd ed. Dubuque, IA: Kendall/Hunt.

Baird, S.M., & Ruth, D.J. (2002). Electronic fetal monitoring of the preterm fetus. *Journal of Perinatal and Neonatal Nursing, 16,* 12–24.

Barrows, H.S., & Tamblyn, R.M. (1980). *Problem based learning: An approach to medical education.* New York: Springer, Inc.

Baskett, T.F., & Liston, R.M. (1989). Fetal movement monitoring: Clinical application. *Clinics in Perinatology, 16,* 613–625.

Benner, P. (1984). *From novice to expert: Excellence and power in clinical nursing practice.* Menlo Park, CA: Addison Wesley, Inc.

Blackburn, S. (2003). *Maternal, fetal & neonatal physiology: A clinical perspective* (pp. 277–291). St Louis, MO: Saunders.

Bobby, P. (2003). Multiple assessment techniques evaluate antepartum fetal risks. *Pediatric Annals, 32* (9), 609–617.

Cabaniss, M. (1993). *Fetal monitoring interpretation.* Philadelphia: Lippincott.

Callen, P. (2000). Amniotic fluid: Its role in fetal health and disease. In P. Callen (Ed.), *Ultrasonography in obstetrics and gynecology* (4th ed.), pp. 638–659. New York: W. B. Saunders.

Centers for Disease Control and Prevention. (2002). Clinical prevention guidelines. Sexually transmitted diseases treatment guidelines 2002. *MMWR: Morbidity and mortality weekly report, 51,* No. RR-6. Retrieved October 29, 2005, from www.cdc.gov/std/treatment/TOC2002TG.htm.

Connors, P.M. (2003). High-risk perinatal issues: Delay in the diagnosis of fetal distress and insufficient documentation. *Journal of Nursing Law, 9,* 19–26.

Cypher, R.L., & Adelsperger, D. (2003). Assessment of fetal oxygenation and acid-base status. In N. Feinstein, K.L. Torgersen, & J. Atterbury (Eds.), *Fetal heart monitoring principles and practices* (3rd ed.), pp. 177–198. Dubuque, IA: Kendall/Hunt.

Cypher, R.L., Adelsperger, D., & Torgersen, K.L. (2003). Interpretation of fetal heart rate patterns. In N. Feinstein, K.L. Torgersen, & J. Atterbury (Eds.), *Fetal heart monitoring principles and practices* (3rd ed.), pp. 113–158. Dubuque, IA: Kendall/Hunt.

Davis, L. (1987). Daily fetal movement counting: A valuable assessment tool. *Journal of Nurse-Midwifery, 32* (1), 11–19.

Dochterman, J.M., & Bulecheck, G.M. (2004). Nursing interventions classification (4th ed). St. Louis, MO: Mosby.

Fedorka, P. (1999). Defining the standard of care. In D.M. Rostant, & R.F. Cady (Eds.) *Liability issues in perinatal nursing* (pp. 23–40). Philadelphia: Lippincott.

Feinstein, N., & Atterbury, J.L. (2003). Intrinsic influences on the fetal heart rate. In N. Feinstein, K.L. Torgersen, & J. Atterbury (Eds.), *Fetal heart monitoring principles and practices* (3rd ed., pp. 39–58). Dubuque, IA: Kendall/Hunt.

Feinstein, N., Torgersen, K.L., & Atterbury, J. (2003). *Fetal heart monitoring principles and practices* (3rd ed.). Dubuque, IA: Kendall/Hunt.

Freeman, R.K., Garite, T.J., & Nageotte, M.P. (2003). *Fetal heart rate monitoring* (3rd ed.). Philadelphia: Lippincott Williams & Wilkins.

Fujioka, S., & Kitaura, Y. (2001). Coxsackie B virus infection in idiopathic dilated cardiomyopathy: Clinical and pharmacological implications. *BioDrugs, 15,* 791–799.

Gaufberg, S. (2004). Abruptio placentae. *eMedicine.* November 24, 2004.

Gegor, C.L., Paine, L.L., & Johnson, T. R. B. (1991). Antepartal fetal assessment: A nurse-midwifery perspective. *Journal of Nurse-Midwifery, 36* (3), 153–167.

Gilbert, E.S., & Harmon, J.S. (2003). *Manual of high-risk pregnancy and delivery* (3rd ed.). St. Louis, MO: Mosby.

Goss, G.L., & Torgersen, K.L. (2003). Extrinsic influences on the fetal heart rate. In N. Feinstein, K.L. Torgersen, & J. Atterbury (Eds.), *Fetal heart monitoring principles and practices* (3rd ed., pp. 25–37). Dubuque, IA: Kendall/Hunt.

Greenwald, L.M., & Mondor, M. (2003). Malpractice and the perinatal nurse. *Journal of Perinatal and Neonatal Nursing, 17,* 101–109.

Harvey, C.J., & Chez, B.F. (1997). *Critical concepts in fetal monitoring* (2nd ed.). Washington, D.C.: Association of Women's Health, Obstetric and Neonatal Nurses.

Hill, G., & Hill, K. (2005). *The people's law dictionary.* Publisher: Fine Communications. Retrieved from the World Wide Web on June 10, 2005.

Joint Commission on Accreditation of Healthcare Organizations. (2004). , Preventing infant death and injury during delivery. *Sentinel Event Alert, Issue 30.* Chicago: Author.

King, T., & Parer, J. (2000). The physiology of fetal heart rate patterns and perinatal asphyxia. *The Journal of Perinatal & Neonatal Nursing, 14,* 19–39.

King, T.L., & Simpson, K.R. (2001). Fetal assessment during labor. In K.R. Simpson & Creehan (Eds.), *Perinatal Nursing* (2nd ed., pp. 378–416). Philadelphia: Lippincott.

King-Urbanski, T., & Cady, R. (1999). Documentation. In D.M. Rostant, & R.F. Cady (Eds.), *Liability issues in perinatal nursing* (pp. 225–241). Philadelphia: Lippincott.

Kleinman, C.S., & Nehgme, R.A. (2004). Cardiac arrhythmias in the human fetus. *Pediatric Cardiology, 25,* 234–251.

Kleinman, C.S., Nehgme, R., & Copel, J.A. (2004). Fetal cardiac arrhythmias. In R.K. Creasy, R. Resnik, & J.D. Iams (Eds.), *Maternal-fetal medicine* (pp. 465–482). Philadelphia: Saunders.

Kontopoulos, E.V., & Vintzileos, A. (2004). Condition specific antepartum fetal testing. *American Journal of Obstetrics and Gynecology, 191,* 1546–1551.

Kühnert, M., and Schimdt, S. (2004). Intrapartum management of nonreassuring fetal heart rate patterns: A randomized controlled trial of fetal pulse oximetry. *American Journal of Obstetrics and Gynecology, 191,* 1989–1995.

Landon, M.B., Catalano, P.M., & Gabbe, S.G. (2002). Diabetes mellitus. In S.G. Gabbe, J.R. Niebyl, & J.L. Simpson (Eds.), *Obstetrics: Normal and problem pregnancies* (4th ed., pp. 1081–1116). New York: Churchill Livingstone.

Larmay, H., & Strasburger, J.F. (2004). Differential diagnosis and management of the fetus and newborn with an irregular or abnormal heart rate. *Pediatric Clinics of North America, 51,* 1033–1050.

Mahley, S., & Beerman, J. (1998). Following the chain of command in an obstetric setting: A nurse's responsibility. *Journal of Legal Nurse Consulting, 9,* 7–13.

Mahoney, K., Torgersen, K.L., & Feinstein, N. (2003). Maternal-fetal assessment. In N. Feinstein, K.L. Torgersen, & J. Atterbury (Eds.), *Fetal heart monitoring principles and practices* (3rd ed., pp. 61–76). Dubuque, IA: Kendall/Hunt.

Manning, F.A., Baskett, T.F., Morrison, I., & Lange, I. (1981). Fetal biophysical scoring: A prospective study in 1,184 high risk patients. *American Journal of Obstetrics and Gynecology, 140,* 289–294.

McCartney, P.R. (2003). Synchronizing with standard time and atomic clocks. *American Journal of Maternal Child Nursing, 28,* 51.

McDonald, B.A. (1990, August). Begin course development with a course blueprint. *Performance and Instruction, 29*(10), 4.

Menihan, C.A., & Zottoli, E.K. (2001). *Electronic fetal monitoring: Concepts and Applications.* New York: Lippincott.

Miller, D.A. (2002). External stimuli. *Clinical Obstetrics and Gynecology, 45,* 1054–1062.

Miller, D.A., Rabello, Y.A., & Paul, R.H. (1996). The modified biophysical profile: Antepartum testing in the 1990s. *American Journal of Obstetrics and Gynecology, 174,* 812–817.

Moffat, F.W., & Feinstein, N. (2003). Techniques for fetal heart assessment. In N. Feinstein, K.L. Torgersen, & J. Atterbury (Eds.), *Fetal heart monitoring principles and practices* (3rd.ed., pp. 77–110). Dubuque, IA: Kendall/Hunt.

National Institute of Child Health and Human Development Research Planning Workshop. (1997). Electronic fetal heart rate monitoring: Research guidelines for interpretation. *Journal of Obstetric, Gynecologic and Neonatal Nursing, 26*(6), 635–640.

National Institutes of Health. (2000). National High Blood Pressure Education Program Working Group on High Blood Pressure in Pregnancy, NIH Publication No. 00-3029. Bethesda, MD: Author.

Oakley, C. (2000). General cardiology: Myocarditis, pericarditis and other pericardial diseases. *Heart 2000, 84,* 449–454.

Olesen, A.G., & Svare, J.A. (2004). Decreased fetal movements: Background, assessment, and clinical management. *Acta Obstetricia et Gynecologica Scandinavica, 83,* 818–826.

Oudijk, M.A., Michon, M.M., Kleinman, C.S., Kapusta, L., Stoutenbeck, P., Visser, G.H., & Meijboom, E.J. (2000). Sotalol in the treatment of fetal dysrhythmias. *Circulation, 101,* 2721-2726.

Pedra, S.R., Smallhorn, J.F., Ryan, G., Chitayat, D., Taylor, G.P., Khan, R., Abdolell, M., & Hornberger, L. (2002). Fetal cardiomyopathies. *Circulation, 106,* 585-591.

Porter, M.L. (2000). Fetal pulse oximetry: An adjunct to electronic fetal heart rate monitoring. *Journal of Obstetric, Gynecologic, and Neonatal Nursing,* 29(5), 537–548.

Ramsay, M.M., James, D.K., Steer, P.J., Weiner, C.P., & Gonik, B. (2000). *Normal Values in Pregnancy,* 2nd ed., (pp. 3–61). London, England: W.B. Saunders.

Rotmensch, S., Liberati, M., Vishne, T. H., Celentano, C., Ben-Rafael, Z, & Bellati, U. (1999). The effects of betamethasone and dexamethasone on fetal heart rate patterns and biophysical activities: A prospective randomized trial. *Acta Obstetricia et Gynecologica Scandinavia, 78,* 493–500.

Royal College of Obstetricians and Gynaecologists. (2001). *The use of electronic fetal monitoring. The use and interpretation of cardiotocography in intrapartum fetal surveillance.* (Evidence-based Clinical Guideline No. 8). Retrieved September 8, 2005 from http://www.rcog.org.uk/resources/public/pdf/efm_guideline_final_2may2001.pdf

Sadovsky, E., & Yaffe, H. (1973). Daily fetal movement recording and fetal prognosis. *Obstetrics & Gynecology, 41,* 845–850.

Schifrin, B.S. (2003). Is fetal pulse oximetry ready for clinical practice?: Writing for the CON position. *American Journal of Maternal Child Nursing,* 28(2), 65.

Schmidt, J.V. (2000). The Development of AWHONN's Fetal Heart Monitoring Principles and Practices Workshop. *Journal of Obstetric, Gynecologic, and Neonatal Nurses,* 29(5), 509–515.

Sibai, B.M. (2002). Hypertension. In S.G. Gabbe, J.R. Niebyl, & J.L. Simpson (Eds.), *Obstetrics: Normal and problem pregnancies.* (4th ed., pp. 945–1004). New York: Churchill Livingstone.

Simpson, J.M., & Sharland, G.K. (1998). Fetal tachycardias: Management and outcome of 127 consecutive cases. *Heart, 79,* 576–581.

Simpson, K.R. (2003). Fetal pulse oximetry update. *Lifelines, 7,* 411–413.

Simpson, K.R. (1998). Fetal oxygen saturation monitoring during labor. *Journal of Perinatal and Neonatal Nursing, 12,* 26–37.

Simpson, K.R. (1998). Using guidelines and standards of care from professional organizations as a framework for competence validation. In K.R. Simpson, & P.A. Creehan (eds.), *Competence Validation for Perinatal Care Providers* (pp. 2–11). Philadelphia: Lippincott.

Simpson, K.R., & Flood Chez, B. (2001). Professional and legal issues. In K.R. Simpson, & P.A. Creehan (eds.), *Perinatal nursing* (2nd ed., pp. 21–52). Philadelphia: Lippincott.

Simpson, K.R., & Creehan, P. A. (Eds.) (2001). *Perinatal nursing* (2nd ed.). Washington, D.C.: Association of Women's Health, Obstetrics, and Neonatal Nursing.

Simpson, K.R., & Knox, F.E. (2003). Communication of fetal heart monitoring information. In K.R. Simpson, & P.A. Creehan (eds.), *Perinatal nursing* (2nd ed., pp. 201–234). Philadelphia: Lippincott.

Simpson, K.R., & James, D. (2005). Efficacy of intrauterine resuscitation techniques in improving fetal oxygen status in labor. *Obstetrics and Gynecology,* 105, 1362–1368.

Simpson, K.R., & Porter, M.L. (2001). Fetal oxygen saturation monitoring: Using this new technology for fetal assessment during labor. *Lifelines,* 5(2), 26–33.

Simpson, K.R., Thorman, K.E., & Ropp, A. (2001). Managing the quality of care. In K.R. Simpson, & P.A. Creehan (eds.), *Perinatal nursing* (2nd ed., pp. 2–20). Philadelphia: Lippincott.

Society of Obstetricians, and Gynaecologists of Canada. (2002a). Fetal health surveillance in labour (SOGC Clinical Practice Guidelines No. 112). *Journal of Obstetrics and Gynaecology in Canada, 112* (March), 1–13.

Sullivan, C.A., & Bowden, M.A. (1999). Nurse-physician communication. In D.M. Rostant, & R.F. Cady (eds.) *Liability issues in perinatal nursing* (pp. 257–270). Philadelphia: Lippincott.

Tekay, A., & Campbell, S. (2000). Doppler ultrasonography in obstetrics. In P. Callen (Ed.), *Ultrasonography in obstetrics and gynecology* (4th ed., pp. 677–723). New York: W.B. Saunders.

Thorp, J.A. (2003). Is fetal pulse oximetry ready for clinical practice? Writing for the PRO position. *American Journal of Maternal Child Nursing, 28*(2), 64.

Torgersen, K. (2003). Fetal arrhythmias and dysrhythmias. In N. Feinstein, K. Torgersen, & J. Atterbury (Eds.), *Fetal heart monitoring principles and practices* (pp. 289–328). Dubuque, IA: Kendall/Hunt.

Trines, J., & Hornberger, L.K. (2004). Evolution of heart disease in utero. *Pediatric Cardiology, 25,* 287–298.

Wilkinson, J. (2005). *Nursing diagnosis handbook* (8th ed.). Upper Saddle River, NJ: Prentice-Hall.

Williams, K.P., Farquharson, D.R., Bebbington, M., Dansereau, J., Galerneau, G., Wilson, R.D., Shaw, D., & Kent, N. (2003). Screening for fetal well-being in a high risk pregnant population comparing the nonstress test with umbilical artery Doppler velocimetry: A randomized controlled clinical trial. *American Journal of Obstetrics and Gynecology, 188* (5), 1366–1371.

Vintzileos, A.M., Campbell, W.A., Ingardia, C.J., & Nochimson, D. (1983). The biophysical profile and its predictive value. *Obstetrics and Gynecology, 62* (2), 271–278.

Vintzileos, A.M., & Hanley, M.L. (2000). Antepartum fetal assessment by ultrasonography: The fetal biophysical profile. In *Ultrasonography in obstetrics and gynecology* (4th ed., pp. 660–676). New York: W.B. Saunders.

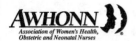

AWHONN
*Association of Women's Health,
Obstetric and Neonatal Nurses*

AWHONN Membership Application

RECRUITED BY   (IF APPLICABLE):

RECRUITER'S MEMBER #:

Membership categories (Choose one)

☐ **Full $149**
RNs licensed in the
US, its territories or
Canada. May hold
elected and appointed
offices and may vote.

☐ **Associate $132**
LPNs, LVNs or others
interested in the health of
women and newborns.
May hold appointed office,
but may not vote.

☐ **Student $75**
Eligible for 4 years.
RNs may vote.
Proof of current
enrollment required.
Please attach.

☐ **Retired $75**
Must be at least 62 and
no longer working as a
nurse. Min. 3 years
previous full membership
required. RNs may vote.

☐ **Disabled $75**
Unable to work.
Statement by
applicant
is acceptable.
RNs may vote.

☐ **International $173**
A nurse or oth er
interested party
residing outside
the US (other than
members of the
US Armed Forces).
RNs may vote.

PREFIX (MS, MR, ETC)   FIRST   MI   LAST   SUFFIX (JR., III, ETC)

CREDENTIALS (RN, CNM, ETC)   TITLE/POSITION (E.G. NURSE MANAGER, MIDWIFE, DIRECTOR, ETC)

HOME ADDRESS   CITY   STATE/PROVINCE

ZIP/POSTAL CODE   COUNTRY   HOME PHONE

EMPLOYER   WORK ADDRESS   CI TY   STATE/PROVINCE   ZIP/POSTAL CODE

WORK PHONE   WORK FAX

PREFERRED E-MAIL ADDRESS FOR AWHONN COMMUNICATION

PREFERRED MAILING ADDRESS (CHECK ONE)   ☐ WORK   ☐ HOME

☐ I AM CURRENTLY AN ACTIVE DUTY MEMBER OF THE US ARMED FORCES. BRANCH OF SERVICE (CHECK ONE)   ☐ ARMY   ☐ NAVY   ☐ AIR FORCE
   (ACTIVE DUTY MEMBERS OF THE US ARMED FORCES WILL BE MEMBERS OF THE AWHONN ARMED FORCES SECTION.)
   RANK :

☐ I AM AFFILIATED WITH THE US ARMED FORCES (RETIRED, RESERVIST, DOD CIVILIAN, ETC) BUT AM NOT ON ACTIVE DUTY, AND I WOULD LIKE TO BE A MEMBER
   OF THE AWHONN ARMED FORCES SECTION INSTEAD OF THE SECTION IN WHICH I RESIDE.

WE OCCASIONALLY MAKE OUR MAILING LIST AVAILABLE TO CAREFULLY SCREENED ORGANIZATIONS THAT OFFER PRODUCTS AND/OR SERVICES THAT MAY BE OF
INTEREST TO YOU. ☐ CHECK THIS BOX ONLY IF YOU DO NOT WANT TO RECEIVE SUCH MAILINGS.

Method of Payment

☐ CHECK OR MONEY ORDER PAYABLE TO AWHONN

☐ VISA   ☐ MASTERCARD   ☐ AMERICAN EXPRESS

CARD NO   EXP DATE

CARD HO LDE R'S NAME

SIGNA TURE

*DUES SUBJECT TO CHANGE. MEMBERSHIP DUES ARE NOT REFUNDABLE.

Amount Enclosed

DUES $

☐ OPTIONAL TAX-DEDUCTIBLE DONATION TO AWHONN   HEALTHFUNDS $20.00

TOTAL E NCLOSED $

ENTER PROMOTI ON CODE HERE, IF ANY

SUBMIT APPLICATION AND PAYMENT TO:
AWHONN, Dept. 4015, Washington, DC 20042-4015

Phone: 800-673-8499; 800-245-0231 (Canada)
Fax: 202-728-0575; www.awhonn.org

Member Profile

We want to make that sure we offer the professional nursing programs, services and products that are of greatest value to you. Please complete this member profile. Your answers will be kept confidential.

IN NURSING PRACTICE SINCE
_____ YEAR ONLY

DATE OF BIRTH
_____ DAY MO YR

GENDER ☐ M ☐ F

Primary Position (select no more than 2)
☐ CASE MANAGER
☐ CLINICAL NURSE SPECIALIST
☐ CONSULTANT
☐ FACULTY-ACADEMIC
☐ NURSE EXECUTIVE
☐ NURSE MANAGER/COORDINATOR
☐ NURSE MIDWIFE
☐ NURSE PRACTITIONER
☐ RESEARCHER
☐ STAFF DEVELOPMENT
☐ STAFF NURSE
☐ STUDENT
☐ OTHER: _____

Ethnic/Racial Background (select one)
☐ AMERICAN INDIAN/ALASKA NATIVE
☐ ASIAN OR PACIFIC ISLANDER
☐ AFRICAN AMERICAN (NON-HISPANIC)
☐ HISPANIC
☐ WHITE (NON-HISPANIC)
☐ MULTIRACIAL

Certifications (check all that apply)
☐ AMBULATORY WOMEN'S HEALTH
☐ CHILDBIRTH EDUCATOR
☐ EFM/FHM
☐ HIGH-RISK OB NURSING
☐ INPATIENT OB
☐ LACTATION CONSULTANT/EDUCATOR
☐ LOW-RISK NEONATAL NURSING
☐ MATERNAL NEWBORN NURSING
☐ NICU NURSING
☐ NEONATAL NURSE PRACTITIONER
☐ NURSING ADMINISTRATION
☐ NURSE MIDWIFE
☐ OB/GYN PRACTITIONER
☐ PERINATAL NURSE PRACTITIONER
☐ PERINATAL NURSING
☐ WOMEN'S HEALTH NURSE PRACTIONER
☐ OTHER: _____

Highest Degree Earned
☐ DOCTORATE
☐ MASTER'S
☐ BACHELOR'S
☐ ASSOCIATE
☐ DIPLOMA
☐ VOC-TECH
☐ OTHER: _____

Medications and/or OTC Products (check all that apply)
☐ HAVE PRESCRIPTIVE AUTHORITY
☐ RECOMMEND MEDICATION AND/OR OTC PRODUCTS
☐ COUNSEL AND EDUCATE PATIENTS REGARDING USE OF MEDICATIONS AND/OR OTC PRODUCTS
☐ NO ROLE REGARDING MEDICATIONS AND/OR OTC PRODUCTS

Equipment and Supplies (check all that apply)
☐ MAKE PURCHASING DECISIONS DIRECTLY
☐ RECOMMEND OR INFLUENCE DECISIONS
☐ NO ROLE REGARDING PURCHASE OF EQUIPMENT AND/OR SUPPLIES

Primary Clinical Focus (select no more than 2)
☐ ANTEPARTUM
☐ BREASTFEEDING/LACTATION
☐ INTRAPARTUM (INCLUDES LDR/LDRP & L&D)
☐ NICU
☐ NURSERY
☐ WOMEN'S HEALTH
☐ POSTPARTUM (INCLUDES MOTHER-BABY)
☐ OTHER: _____

Job Setting
☐ ACADEMIA
☐ AMBULATORY CARE (INCLUDES PHYSICIAN OFFICE, OUTPATIENT CLINIC, ETC.)
☐ HOME HEALTH CARE
☐ HOSPITAL INPATIENT
☐ NOT WORKING
☐ PUBLIC HEALTH
☐ SELF-EMPLOYED
☐ OTHER: _____

Majority of Time Spent (select no more than 2)
☐ ADMINISTRATION
☐ CONSULTING
☐ DIRECT PATIENT CARE
☐ MANAGEMENT/SUPERVISION
☐ PATIENT EDUCATION
☐ RESEARCH
☐ STAFF DEVELOPMENT/EDUCATION
☐ UNDERGRAD/GRADUATE NURSING EDUCATION
☐ OTHER: _____

Is Continuing Education (CE) required for you to maintain licensure and/or certification?
☐ YES   ☐ NO

Other memberships
☐ AACN (CRITICAL CARE NURSES) ☐ AANP ☐ ACNM ☐ ANA ☐ ANN ☐ AONE ☐ NANN ☐ NPWH ☐ SIGMA THETA TAU
☐ OTHER: _____

How did you learn about AWHONN?
☐ COLLEAGUE
☐ ADVERTISEMENT
☐ MAILING
☐ CONFERENCE/CONVENTION
☐ OTHER: _____

SUBMIT APPLICATION AND PAYMENT TO:
AWHONN, Dept. 4015, Washington, DC 20042-4015

Phone: 800-673-8499; 800-245-0231 (Canada)
Fax: 202-728-0575; www.awhonn.org

ADVANCED FETAL MONITORING COURSE
TEST B ANSWER SHEET

Participant Name: _____

Test B is to be administered only if the participant does not successfully complete Test A. If the participant successfully completes Test B, Competence Validation will be awarded. If the participants fails both Test A and Test B, Competence Validation should not be awarded.

Each participant should keep his/her copy of the test booklet and Test B results. The corresponding original questions should be retained by the instructor. This form should not be mailed back to the AWHONN processing center.

Answer Sheet

A B C	A B C	A B C	A B C	A B C
1 ○ ○ ○	11 ○ ○ ○	21 ○ ○ ○	31 ○ ○ ○	41 ○ ○ ○
2 ○ ○ ○	12 ○ ○ ○	22 ○ ○ ○	32 ○ ○ ○	42 ○ ○ ○
3 ○ ○ ○	13 ○ ○ ○	23 ○ ○ ○	33 ○ ○ ○	43 ○ ○ ○
4 ○ ○ ○	14 ○ ○ ○	24 ○ ○ ○	34 ○ ○ ○	44 ○ ○ ○
5 ○ ○ ○	15 ○ ○ ○	25 ○ ○ ○	35 ○ ○ ○	45 ○ ○ ○
6 ○ ○ ○	16 ○ ○ ○	26 ○ ○ ○	36 ○ ○ ○	46 ○ ○ ○
7 ○ ○ ○	17 ○ ○ ○	27 ○ ○ ○	37 ○ ○ ○	47 ○ ○ ○
8 ○ ○ ○	18 ○ ○ ○	28 ○ ○ ○	38 ○ ○ ○	48 ○ ○ ○
9 ○ ○ ○	19 ○ ○ ○	29 ○ ○ ○	39 ○ ○ ○	49 ○ ○ ○
10 ○ ○ ○	20 ○ ○ ○	30 ○ ○ ○	40 ○ ○ ○	50 ○ ○ ○

STUDY GUIDE

Advanced Fetal Monitoring Review

Preparation for Advanced Fetal Monitoring Course

1 © 2006 AWHONN

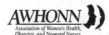

This self-study is designed as a **prerequisite to the Advanced Fetal Monitoring Course (AFMC) and provides a core review of key principles of fetal monitoring. It is imperative that you have a working knowledge of the information contained in this self-study prior to taking the AFMC.** In preparation for your participation in the Advanced Fetal Monitoring Course, it is necessary for you to understand fundamental information used in fetal heart monitoring (FHM). Since you are an experienced clinician, some of this information may be a review, but new aspects are also included. To streamline the AFMC and make it more interactive and interesting to you, this information is provided to you in a self-study format. **Your participation in the workshop will be enhanced by your completion of this study packet *prior* to your attendance at the AFMC.** This review may also enhance your clinical decision making. Your understanding of the information provided will also allow you to participate more fully in the workshop. **Please be aware that the information contained in this self-study will be included in the competency evaluation test given at the conclusion of the course.**

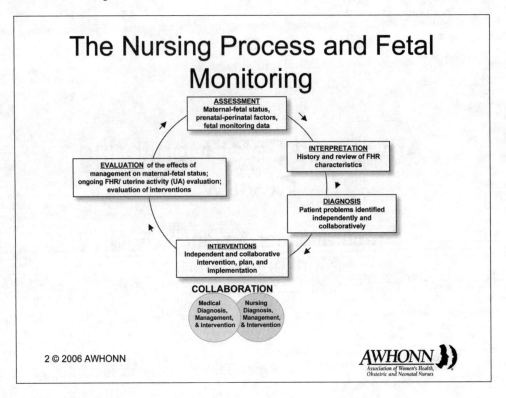

The nursing process model pictured on this slide was created for the original AWHONN FHMPP workshop (Feinstein, Torgersen & Atterbury, 2003). It provides the theoretical framework for the FHMPP and AFMC course and the textbook. The model highlights steps of the critical thinking process related to fetal heart monitoring and should be viewed as a problem-solving process represented by a continuum of assessment, interpretation, diagnosis, intervention, evaluation and collaboration among health care providers.

- **First, you perform a comprehensive initial assessment.**
- **You then combine the assessment information with your knowledge and experience to analyze and interpret the clinical situation.** It is important in this step that you examine the whole clinical picture and determine how the pieces of the data gathered interact with each other. It is also important that you base your assessment and interventions on the underlying physiology to help prioritize and plan care appropriately.
- **Individualized nursing diagnoses are developed from this interpretation and will guide your interventions.** The interventions are based on physiological goals. These diagnoses and interventions may be independent or collaborative.
- **Next, you evaluate your interventions to determine if your goals have been met.** If not, the process is repeated.
- Notice how the steps move in a circular motion and are never-ending. The intrapartum period is dynamic; therefore subsequent assessments will direct this ongoing nursing process. Decision making relating to fetal heart monitoring (FHM) data is based on critical thinking skills and their application to the nursing process.

Nursing Database

History
- Family
- Medical-surgical
- Obstetric
- Psychosocial

Current Pregnancy
- Medical-surgical
- Obstetric
- Psychosocial
- Support

Patient Interview

Physical Assessment

3 © 2006 AWHONN

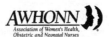

AWHONN
Association of Women's Health,
Obstetric and Neonatal Nurses

A comprehensive approach is important when performing the initial assessment. As you can see on this slide, this approach includes **gathering data from the woman's history, including family, medical-surgical, obstetric and psychosocial issues. You should also assess medical-surgical, obstetric or psychosocial issues and concerns during the woman's current pregnancy, including the presence and quality or absence of support persons. A confidential patient interview and complete physical assessment will provide the information needed to establish your nursing database (Mahoney, Torgersen, & Feinstein, 2003).**

The patient's stated physical and/or emotional needs typically guide the assessment process. For instance, if the woman arrives stating she feels an urge to push, your initial assessment would focus on determining if the patient is delivering imminently and, if so, then preparing for delivery. On the other hand, your assessment may uncover information that is unrelated to the woman's expressed need and that may then become a top priority. For example, a patient may arrive complaining of uterine contractions. Upon further assessment, if she is found to have absent fetal heart tones, that data would require immediate further investigation and notification of the primary care provider; as well as provision of information and emotional support for the woman and her partner.

Nursing Database (Cont.)

Purpose of comprehensive patient assessment:

- Identify normal findings
- Identify risk factors that may affect maternal-fetal status
- Risk assessment influences maternal-fetal nursing care

4 © 2006 AWHONN

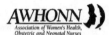

AWHONN))
Association of Women's Health,
Obstetric and Neonatal Nurses

It is critical to include a review of the patient's prenatal records, a patient interview and complete head-to-toe physical assessment to establish a nursing database. This database allows us to identify and confirm normal findings or risk factors. The risk assessment will play a lead role in your critical thinking and implementation of the nursing process on a continuum. This procedure may need to be abbreviated in an emergent situation with a focus on gathering data pertinent to the immediate situation. Reliance on verbal reports may be necessary initially, but it is essential to gather the complete information when possible.

- **What are some examples of risk factors commonly identified for intrapartum patients?**
  Preeclampsia, postdates, intrauterine growth restriction (IUGR), diabetes, cigarette smoking, genetic factors, young maternal age, substance abuse, etc.
- After completing the risk assessment, as you can see on the slide, next you should think about how this will influence your nursing care for this woman.
- **What are some examples of how risk factors could affect the maternal-fetal status and our nursing care?**
  Decreased placental functioning capacity, increased risk for fetal anomalies, oligohydramnios, decreased fetal movement, lack of coping mechanisms and/or support system, etc. Your nursing care will focus on being alert for clinical information that may be associated with these factors.
- **Let's use an example: A patient admitted for an induction for oligohydramnios and intrauterine growth restriction (IUGR) is at risk for what potential physiologic problems?**
  Cord compression and/or uteroplacental insufficiency.
- **What nursing diagnoses can we create for this woman?**

Sample Nursing Diagnoses

- Risk for impaired fetal gas exchange related to umbilical cord compression secondary to oligohydramnios

- Risk for ineffective fetal tissue perfusion related to uteroplacental perfusion insufficiency secondary to inadequate placental function.

5 © 2006 AWHONN

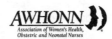

Two possible nursing diagnoses are:

- **Risk for impaired fetal gas exchange related to umbilical cord compression secondary to oligohydramnios.**
- **Risk for ineffective fetal tissue perfusion related to uteroplacental perfusion insufficiency secondary to inadequate placental function.**

Can you think of others?

For this type of patient, your main concerns are the increased risks for cord compression and/or decreased uteroplacental perfusion. Nursing interventions should address these concerns. Your interventions could include maintaining optimal uterine blood flow and umbilical circulation with lateral maternal positioning and hydration, as well as intrapartum fetal heart monitoring.

Your nursing diagnoses and nursing care, then, should reflect that you appreciate the patient's increased risk for what kind of fetal heart rate (FHR) characteristics? Variable and late decelerations and possibly decreased variability, depending on the patient's individual circumstances. You would monitor for these FHR changes and intervene appropriately.

Extrinsic Factors

- Extrinsic factors:
  - Influences outside the fetus that affect O2 availability to the fetus & can affect FHR
- Extrinsic factors include:
  - Maternal oxygen transport
  - Uterine blood flow
  - Placental integrity
  - Umbilical blood flow

6 © 2006 AWHONN

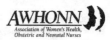

Let's now discuss extrinsic factors and their possible effects on the FHR.

Extrinsic factors are influences outside of the fetus that affect the *availability of oxygen to the fetus,* thus affecting the FHR (Goss & Torgersen, 2003).

As you can see on the slide, **maternal oxygen transport** is one part of the group of extrinsic factors that can influence the fetal heart rate. Maternal oxygen transport will be discussed in the AFMC.

Others are: **blood flow to the uterus, integrity of the placenta and the flow of blood through the cord.**

In our later discussion on interventions, you will see that oftentimes our interventions will affect one or more of these extrinsic factors, thus affecting the availability of oxygen to the fetus and potentially the fetal heart rate or pattern.

Let's take a closer look at the extrinsic factors.

Uterine Blood Flow

- Supplied by maternal spiral arteries extending through myometrium & endometrium
- Spiral arteries dilate in pregnancy to ↑ uterine blood flow
- Blood supply to placenta is dependant on adequate uterine blood flow

7 © 2006 AWHONN

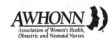

Our discussion of extrinsic factors begins with uterine blood flow. First, it is important to understand how blood is supplied to the uterus.

- **Uterine blood flow is supplied through the maternal spiral arteries.** These arteries extend perpendicularly through the myometrium and endometrium, so contraction of uterine muscles compresses these arteries (King & Parer, 2000). Compression of the uterine arteries with contractions may adversely affect oxygenation of the fetus.
- Another interesting fact about maternal spiral arteries is a process that takes place in early placental development. **These tightly coiled arteries in a nonpregnant uterus should become widely dilated vessels in early pregnancy, thus accommodating the large increase in blood flow during pregnancy.** This process becomes clinically important because it causes the spiral arteries to lose their ability to autoregulate, or constrict if their internal pressure drops. *The blood supply to the placenta, then, is totally dependent on adequate blood flow to the uterus.*
- **At times, the spiral arteries remain tightly coiled, therefore the blood flow to the placenta may be inadequate.** This may cause a failure to meet the needs of a growing fetus (King & Parer, 2000).

Extrinsic Factors (cont.)

Uterine blood flow facilitated by:

- maintaining maternal lateral position or lateral tilt
- ensuring adequate maternal hydration
- enhancing maternal relaxation
- providing appropriate pain management

8 © 2006 AWHONN

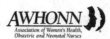

As was mentioned on the previous slide, the blood flow to the placenta is totally dependent on adequate blood flow to the uterus. A variety of routine interventions can enhance uterine blood flow.

What are some ways we can and should do this?

Maintaining maternal lateral position whenever possible, or ensuring a lateral tilt to avoid the supine position

- **Ensuring adequate maternal hydration**

- **Enhancing maternal relaxation by providing labor support and comfort measures**

- **Providing appropriate pain management (Goss & Torgersen, 2003):**

Conversely, there are factors that may decrease blood flow to the uterus.
Can you think of some examples?

Extrinsic Factors (cont.)

Uterine blood flow can be inhibited by:

- Supine positioning
- Maternal stress or exercise
- Uterine contractions
- Maternal hypotension
- Maternal hypertension

(Goss & Torgersen, 2003; Freeman, 2003)

9 © 2006 AWHONN

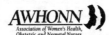

Uterine blood flow can be decreased by many factors (Goss & Torgersen, 2003; Freeman, 2003):

- **Supine positioning**–compression of maternal great vessels may cause decreased venous return and decreased blood flow to the uterus
- **Maternal stress or exercise**–may divert blood away from uterus
- **Uterine contractions**–compression of uterine vessels
- **Maternal hypotension from anesthesia or hypovolemia as examples**–decreased blood flow to uterus
- **Maternal hypertension**–decreased blood flow to uterus and placenta

Certain medication may also affect uterine blood flow. These will be discussed throughout the course.

- The fetus may respond to decreased uterine blood flow by exhibiting particular fetal heart rate patterns. It is important to consider uterine blood flow and its effects on the oxygenation of the fetus when caring for your patients. Interventions should be directed to maximize uterine blood flow.
- Remember that uterine blood flow is important because it affects blood supply to the placenta, about 70-90% of the blood flow to the uterus passes through the intervillous spaces of the placenta (Goss & Torgersen, 2003).

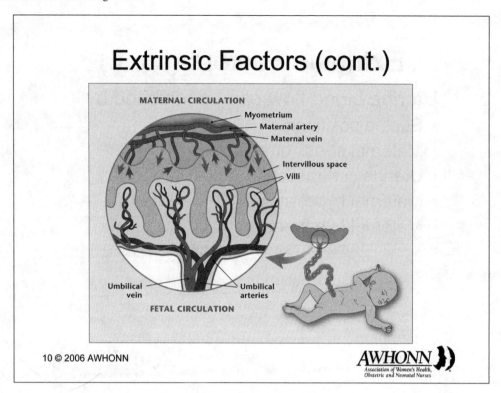

The placenta functions as the fetus's lungs, kidneys, and gastrointestinal and integumentary systems. It also functions as a protective barrier to the fetus and an endocrine organ by releasing hormones (Freeman, 2003). The placental function focus for this class will be fetal oxygenation, since the purpose of continuous electronic FHR monitoring is to assess the fetal oxygenation status.

- The maternal side of the placenta at term is made up of 15 to 20 cotyledons or lobules. Within each cotyledon is a unit of maternal-fetal circulation. As we look closely at this picture of the placental structure, we can see from the center portion of our picture that the maternal arterial blood is pumped at high pressures into the intervillous space. The forceful presence of the arterial blood, with a mean arterial pressure (MAP) of approximately 90 mmHg, encourages the passive return of fetal oxygen-poor blood into the lower pressures of the maternal venous system (Goss & Torgersen, 2003).
- On the fetal side, each lobule contains the branches of a single large main stem villus.
- The maternal and fetal circulations are separated by two layers—the fetal connective tissue within the branches of the villus and the fetal capillary wall (Freeman, 2003).
- The intervillous space serves as the means for maternal-fetal transfer of oxygen, carbon dioxide (CO_2), nutrients and waste products. Oxygen and CO_2 exchange occurs by the method of passive diffusion (substances pass from gradients of high to low concentration) (Goss & Torgersen, 2003).

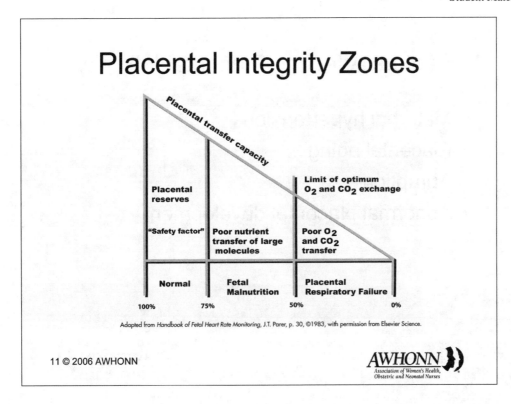

Placental Integrity Zones

Placental transfer capacity

		Limit of optimum O_2 and CO_2 exchange
Placental reserves		
"Safety factor"	Poor nutrient transfer of large molecules	Poor O_2 and CO_2 transfer
Normal	Fetal Malnutrition	Placental Respiratory Failure
100%	75%	50% 0%

Adapted from *Handbook of Fetal Heart Rate Monitoring*, J.T. Parer, p. 30, ©1983, with permission from Elsevier Science.

11 © 2006 AWHONN

AWHONN))
Association of Women's Health, Obstetric and Neonatal Nurses

The integrity of the placenta and the blood supply to the placenta are extremely important! Anything that decreases the effective surface area of the placenta and/or the blood supply to the placenta will increase the potential for fetal malnutrition and potentially decrease oxygen delivery to the fetus.

- This slide illustrates the effects of placental transfer capacity on the limits of fetal transfer of nutrients, O_2 and CO_2.
- As you can see here, at a transfer capacity near 100%, the fetus is supplied with approximately twice the resources to meet its needs.
- When the transfer capacity decreases to around 75%, the transfer of the larger nutrient molecules are affected, and fetal malnutrition can result, potentially leading to intrauterine growth restriction (IUGR).
- At a transfer capacity of approximately 50%, O_2 and CO_2 exchange is decreased, which can result in significant fetal compromise.

Factors Affecting Placental Integrity:

- Maternal hypertension
- Placental aging
- Abruption
- Abnormal placental development

12 © 2006 AWHONN

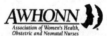

When you perform your assessments and assign risk factors to patients, consider conditions that may affect the integrity of the placenta.

What are some factors that can affect the integrity of the placenta?

- **Maternal hypertension**–constriction of maternal vessels may decrease blood flow to the placenta. This can cause infarcts of the placenta, thus decreasing the functioning placental surface area.
- **Placental aging** can cause calcifications which, again, may decrease the functioning placental surface area.
- **Abruption** will also decrease the functional placental surface area. The amount of the abruption will determine the amount of placental surface area affected.
- **Abnormal placental development,** such as extrachorial placentation, circummarginate and circumvillate placentas, and inadequate lengthening of maternal spiral arteries (which we previously discussed) can also have an effect on placental function (Harvey & Chez, 1997).
- You should consider each patient's placental function and observe fetal heart rate data for information indicating the possibility of poor placental function.

What FHR might indicate decreased placental function?

We would most likely see abnormal baseline ranges, late decelerations and/or absent FHR variability.

Extrinsic Factors (cont.)

Umbilical cord integrity affected by:

- Structural defects
- Cord compression
- Cord cushioning

13 © 2006 AWHONN

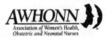

Blood flow through the umbilical cord is the last extrinsic factor we will examine.

The umbilical cord at term is approximately 50 to 60 cm long. It contains three vessels: one umbilical vein carrying oxygenated blood to the fetus, and two umbilical arteries carrying deoxygenated blood away from the fetus. These vessels are surrounded by a protecting substance called Wharton's jelly (Harvey & Chez, 1997).

- Blood must flow freely through the cord to maximize oxygen delivery to the fetus. If the blood is not able to flow freely through the umbilical cord, you may see changes in the FHR.
- **What changes would you most likely see?** Variable decelerations.
- The assessment of the **fetal tolerance** to decreased umbilical blood flow should include an assessment of the entire clinical situation with the FHR response. Clinical interventions can then be made based on those assessments in collaboration with other team members.
- **Umbilical blood flow can be affected by** (Goss & Torgersen, 2003; Harvey & Chez, 1997):
  - **Structural abnormalities** such as a velementous insertion, decreased number of vessels in the cord or hematomas
  - **Cord compression** caused by mechanical conditions such as maternal/fetal position in relation to cord location, loops of cord wrapped around parts of the fetal body or cord prolapse
  - **Cord cushioning** affected by decreased amounts of amniotic fluid and/or Wharton's jelly

Intrinsic Factors

- Fetal oxygen transport
- Fetal circulation
- Fetal nervous system
- Baroreceptors
- Chemoreceptors
- Hormones
- Fetal reserves
- Fetal homeostatic mechanisms

(Feinstein & Atterbury, 2003)

14 © 2006 AWHONN

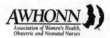

Let's now shift our attention to intrinsic factors affecting fetal oxygenation and the fetal heart rate. Intrinsic factors are those factors found within the fetal body that provide for oxygenation, growth and responses when fetal physiology is stressed. They include (Feinstein & Atterbury, 2003):

- **Fetal oxygen transport**
- **Fetal circulation**
- **Fetal nervous system**
- **Baroreceptors**
- **Chemoreceptors**
- **Hormones**
- **Fetal reserves**
- **Fetal homeostatic mechanisms**

Fetal Nervous System

- Autonomic Nervous System
  - Parasympathetic: ↓ FHR
  - Sympathetic: ↑ FHR
- Chemoreceptors detect changes in gasses
- Baroreceptors detect changes in pressure
- Hormones are secreted in response to hypoxemia

15 © 2006 AWHONN

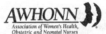

The first intrinsic factor we will discuss affecting the fetal heart rate is the fetal nervous system. This should be familiar information, but it is always important to review as primary fetal heart regulation physiology.

The two branches of the autonomic nervous system exert opposing influences on the FHR. Parasympathetic, or vagus nerve stimulation, decreases the heart rate. Sympathetic stimulation, through nerve fibers widely distributed on the fetal myocardium, will increase the fetal heart rate.

Chemoreceptors and baroreceptors are other intrinsic factors. Chemoreceptors detect biochemical changes in the fetal blood stream, such as changes in the pH, O_2 or CO_2. Baroreceptors detect changes in the fetal blood pressure (Feinstein & Atterbury, 2003).

The parasympathetic and sympathetic branches respond to the messages sent from chemoreceptors and baroreceptors to increase or decrease the heart rate according to the message received (Harvey & Chez, 1997).

For example, fetal hypoxemia (decreased O_2 in the blood) will be detected by the chemoreceptors. **A message will then be sent through the Central Nervous System (CNS) by the release of specific hormones to the sympathetic nervous system to increase the heart rate.**

Hormones

- Catecholamines
  - Epinephrine
  - Norepinephrine
- Vasopressin
- Renin-angiotensin

16 © 2006 AWHONN

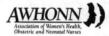

Let's take a closer look at the hormones and their specific functions.

The hormones-another intrinsic influence-function as the messengers. The hormones tell each player what to do.

Examples of hormones that influence the FHR are listed on this slide. Let's discuss the roles of these hormones.

Catecholamines: The release of **epinephrine and norepinephrine** will cause an increase in the FHR and peripheral vasoconstriction. A stimulus that will cause their release is oxygen deprivation. Release of catecholamines will cause blood to be shunted toward the vital organs; the brain, heart and adrenals in the fetus, and decrease blood flow to the periphery. For example, gastrointestinal and renal blood flow.

Vasopressin: This antidiuretic hormone will result in an increase in blood pressure and stabilization of the hemodynamic system.

Renin-angiotensin: It is released by the kidneys to produce vasoconstriction to minimize blood pressure changes in the fetus (Feinstein & Atterbury, 2003).

We know that the maturity of these systems is gestational age dependent. An immature fetus will not have the ability to respond to stressors like a mature fetus. It is thus very important to take into account the fetus's gestational age when assessing fetal well-being from an electronic FHR tracing.

Intrinsic Compensatory Response

Hypoxemia

↓

Chemoreceptor/Baroreceptor stimulation

↓

Neurohormonal responses, including catecholamine production

↓

↓ peripheral and ↑ central organ blood flow

↓

FHR changes

17 © 2006 AWHONN

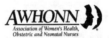

AWHONN
*Association of Women's Health,
Obstetric and Neonatal Nurses*

- The previous slide explained the fetal response of shunting blood toward the vital organs when there is decreased oxygenation. Because of these responses, a healthy fetus can maintain aerobic metabolism under conditions that produce transient decreases in oxygen availability. Examples of these conditions may include supine positioning, uterine contractions and/or intermittent cord compression.
- **The ability of the fetus to maintain this aerobic metabolism is accomplished by the redistribution of blood to the vital organs—the brain, heart, and adrenals, as depicted in this slide.** With the release of catecholamines, and the resulting peripheral vasoconstriction, blood is directed away from the periphery. The peripheral vasoconstriction also causes blood to be shunted toward the brain, heart and adrenals. Thus, the fetus may survive periods of decreased oxygenation without damage to its vital organs (King & Parer, 2000).

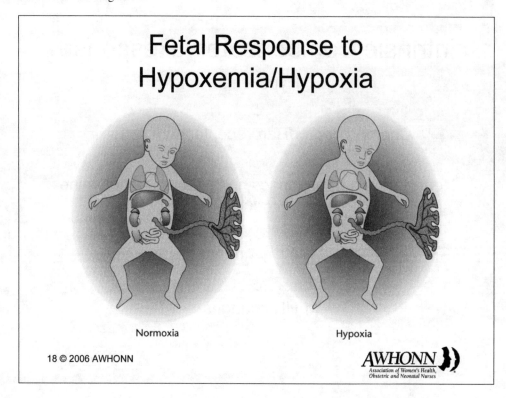

- Episodes of decreased oxygenation may occur abruptly, such as in the case of placental abruption or umbilical cord prolapse. They can also occur intermittently as with uterine contractions or maternal exercise.
- For example, in a fetus with a nuchal cord, initially you may see typical variable decelerations occurring with uterine contractions. However, if the uterine activity is excessive and/or if the labor is prolonged, the FHR pattern may evolve into tachycardia, with atypical variable deceleration characteristics and/or minimal/absent variability.
- If episodes of decreased oxygenation occur chronically, such as with preeclampsia or smoking, or if there is chronic malnourishment of the fetus, the fetal response of shunting blood toward the vital organs will be ongoing. The result may be asymmetrical intrauterine growth restriction (IUGR) with more growth and development of the areas containing the vital organs (head and chest) and less growth and development of the abdomen and periphery. This is sometimes called *brain-sparing* and the newborn may look like the one pictured on the right side of the slide.
- The type of insult may be reflected in the characteristics of the fetal heart rate patterns (Feinstein & Atterbury, 2003; King & Parer, 2000).

Examples of Fetal Responses to Hypoxemia/Hypoxia

- Oligohydramnios
- Gradual hypoxia effect
- Intrauterine growth restriction (IUGR)

19 © 2006 AWHONN

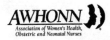

Fetal responses to hypoxemia or hypoxia can also include those that are evident outside of FHR changes. These may include:

- **Oligohydramnios**–In the absence of abnormal fetal kidney function, can be the result of chronic hypoxia and its result of distribution of blood away from nonvital organs, including the kidneys (Vintzileos & Hanley, 2000).
- **Gradual hypoxia effect**–Biophysical activities that appear first in fetal life are the last to disappear during fetal hypoxia. This means that the parameters of FHR reactivity (early third trimester) and fetal breathing movements (~21 weeks), which are the last to develop, will become compromised first with the presence of acidemia (<7.20). With advancing acidemia (>7.10<7.20), fetal body movements (~9 weeks) and fetal tone (~7.5-8.5 weeks) will decrease. And when the acidemia progresses to <7.10, fetal body movements and fetal tone will become absent (Vintzileos & Hanley, 2000). This will be further discussed in the AFHMPP Workshop.
- **IUGR** may also be apparent as a result of chronic hypoxia and the resultant redistribution of blood to the vital organs (Feinstein, et al., 2003).
- The fetal response to hypoxemia and/or hypoxia depends on the degree and duration of the insult. The tolerance of a specific fetus to varying degrees and durations of insults will depend on its fetal reserve.

Fetal Reserve

The degree of hypoxemia that the fetus can tolerate before true tissue hypoxia and acidosis occur.

(Feinstein & Atterbury, 2003)

20 © 2006 AWHONN

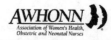

- Fetal reserve is defined as **the degree of hypoxemia that the fetus can tolerate before true tissue hypoxia and acidosis occur** (Feinstein & Atterbury, 2003).
- You will recall from our discussion about the integrity of the placenta that a healthy well-nourished and well-oxygenated fetus is supplied with approximately two times the resources that it needs to thrive and grow.
- The tissue requirement of the fetus is typically less than the resources delivered. This reserve allows the fetus to withstand temporary changes in oxygen supply that are common during labor. When O_2 supply is decreased, preferential blood flow to the vital organs can allow the fetus to compensate for periods of transient hypoxemia, such as commonly occur during labor. This process of preferential blood distribution can also occur in a chronic state of decreased oxygen and/or nutrition to the fetus. This allows growth and development of the vital organs, such as the brain, heart and adrenals. These fetuses, though, may show an intolerance to stress, such as labor, because of inadequate fetal reserves.

Fetal Reserve (cont.)

Present Fetal Reserve	**Decreased Fetal Reserve**
• Normal baseline range	• Abnormal baseline range
• Accelerations	• No accelerations
• Moderate variability	• Minimal/absent variability
• No decelerations	• Decelerations

21 © 2006 AWHONN

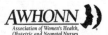

AWHONN
Association of Women's Health,
Obstetric and Neonatal Nurses

- Think of fetal reserves as a gas tank. A healthy fetus will come to labor with a full tank of gas, on which it can rely to meet its needs during labor. A fetus that has been chronically stressed may not have enough gas in its tank to rely on during labor. Then again, some fetuses will not have any gas because they have had to use all of their supplies of oxygen and/or nutrients. Or, they may not have been supplied with the extra resources that they usually need.
- You may see fetal heart rate characteristics that indicate the presence or absence of fetal reserve. **What patterns would indicate the presence of fetal reserve (or a full tank of gas)?**
  - A normal baseline range, moderate variability, no decelerations and, certainly, accelerations
- **What patterns could indicate a possibly diminished fetal reserve (or an empty tank of gas)?**
  - Minimal or absent variability, late decelerations, absence of accelerations
- One of our continual assessments during labor is that of the presence/absence of fetal reserve. How much gas does this fetus have?

Let's briefly review the tools of FHR monitoring that we can use to help us assess the presence or absence of fetal reserve.

Techniques for Monitoring

Indirect	Direct
FHR Fetoscope Ultrasound Transducer (US)	**FHR** Spiral Electrode (SE)
Uterine Activity Palpation Tocotransducer (TOCO)	**Uterine Activity** Intrauterine Pressure Catheter (IUPC)

22 © 2006 AWHONN

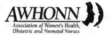

It is necessary in the process of fetal heart monitoring interpretation that the practitioner know the different techniques available to assess the FHR and uterine activity (UA).

These are listed on the slide:

The FHR can be assessed by a fetoscope, an ultrasound transducer or a fetal spiral electrode. Uterine activity can be assessed by palpation, a tocotransducer or an intrauterine pressure catheter.

- It is also important to know how each method works and its benefits and limitations. A thorough review is in the FHMPP textbook.
- Clinical decisions can be made regarding the method of monitoring according to the information that is needed in a particular clinical situation.
- When deciding on whether direct, or more invasive techniques are necessary, you should consider whether the added information received is worth the added risk of introducing an internal device.
- It is also necessary to know troubleshooting techniques for each device in case problems occur during monitoring.

Assessment and Interpretation

Fetal Heart Rate

- Baseline
- Variability
- Periodic/Episodic changes

Uterine Activity

- Frequency
- Duration
- Intensity
- Resting tone

23 © 2006 AWHONN

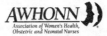
AWHONN
Association of Women's Health,
Obstetric and Neonatal Nurses

- Again, since you are experienced in FHR tracing interpretation, our discussion of FHR patterns and uterine activity assessment will be brief. More information can be found in the FHMPP textbook.
- FHR assessment includes an evaluation of:
  - **Baseline**
  - **Variability**
  - **Periodic/Nonperiodic changes**
- Uterine activity assessment includes an evaluation of:
  - **Frequency**
  - **Duration**
  - **Intensity**
  - **Resting tone**
- When assessing uterine activity, you should consider what effect the UA has on the FHR. It is also essential, in each clinical situation, to consider whether the UA is appropriate or excessive.
- With each assessment, a decision is made whether the FHR and uterine activity interpretation, along with its application to the entire clinical picture, is reassuring or nonreassuring. Then interventions can be made according to the applicable physiologic goals. Let's first talk some more about your decisions based on assessments.

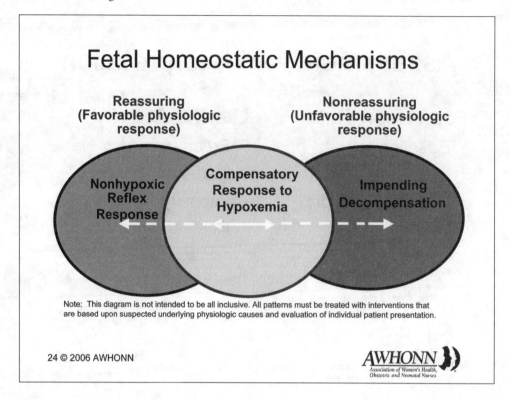

Fetal status frequently changes according to its intrinsic response to extrinsic factors. Ultimately, you will decide whether you are reassured or not by information you have gathered related to maternal-fetal status. **The illustration seen on this slide represents the changes that may occur with their possible resulting FHR pattern.**

- You may see a **nonhypoxic reflex response,** such as an **acceleration.** This is a favorable, or reassuring, response. The nurse could interpret this type of tracing, taking into account the entire clinical picture, as **"green light."** The interpretation of this tracing is reassuring; physiologic goals are being met.
- You may also see a **compensatory response to hypoxemia,** such as those seen in the middle, yellow circle. A typical **variable deceleration** would be an example of this. Tracings that fall into this category could be called **"yellow light." Interventions should be directed to meet physiologic goals and hopefully shift the FHR pattern to "green light."**
- The tracing could also have characteristics that are included in the **red circle. This fetus may be exhibiting signs of impending decompensation, such as repetitive late decelerations,** and be categorized as **"red light."** Interventions, again, would be made to maximize physiologic goals, but realize these fetuses may no longer be able to compensate especially if the situation cannot be corrected or if the fetus has been in the "red light" zone for an extended period of time, leading to a loss of fetal compensatory mechanisms (Feinstein, Torgersen & Atterbury, 2003).
- **Notice on the slide how the arrows move between the circles and how they overlap.** That is because the labor process is a very dynamic time, and FHR patterns will change according to the clinical situation.
- Some tracings may not exhibit characteristics that are easily interpreted or defined-they may not fit into a category listed in this illustration. **If the tracing causes confusion, it should be investigated further in collaboration with other members of the team of care providers.**
- As the tracing exhibits features that are exhibited further to the right in this illustration, the concern about adequacy of oxygenation of the fetus should increase.

Interventions

- Based on physiology
- Four physiological goals
  - Maximize utero-placental blood flow
  - Maximize umbilical circulation
  - Maximize oxygenation
  - Reduce uterine activity

25 © 2006 AWHONN

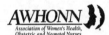

Determining appropriate interventions for observed FHR patterns and clinical situations requires us to integrate the information we have gathered, including our nursing database, initial and subsequent assessment data, interpretations of FHR and UA patterns and their relating physiology. We must examine the relationship between the pieces of information and decide the appropriate interventions.

These interventions are based on four physiologic goals:

- **Maximize utero-placental blood flow**
- **Maximize umbilical circulation**
- **Maximize oxygenation**
- **Reduce uterine activity**

It is important to consider the underlying physiology when determining what goals should be targeted in a clinical situation. The goals help guide you from assessment to intervention.

Let's take a closer look at specific interventions targeted toward these goals.

Maximize Utero-Placental Blood Flow

- Maternal lateral position
- Hydration
- Medication
- Anxiety reduction

26 © 2006 AWHONN

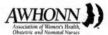

By maximizing uterine blood flow, we can increase the oxygen delivery to the placental/fetal unit. Interventions to maximize utero-placental blood flow may include those shown on this slide.

Maternal position change
Hydration
Medication
Anxiety reduction

How might changing the maternal position maximize uterine blood flow?

- By avoiding the maternal supine position, you will prevent compression of the abdominal aorta and vena cava so cardiac return and cardiac output will be maximized.
- **Hydration** will potentially maximize intravascular volume.
- **Medications,** such as a tocolytic, will reduce uterine activity, thus enhancing utero-placental blood flow. A reduction or discontinuance of uterotonic medications may have a similar effect.
- **Anxiety and/or pain reduction** measures may reduce the release of catecholamines which cause blood to be shunted away from the uterus.
- **What FHR characteristics might indicate the need to address this goal?**
  Absent or minimal variability; late decelerations, prolonged decelerations

Maximize Umbilical Circulation

- Maternal position change
- Elevation of presenting part
- Amnioinfusion

27 © 2006 AWHONN

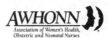

What type of FHR pattern may indicate a need to address this goal?
Variable decelerations

What are some interventions that may maximize umbilical blood flow?

- **A change in the mother's position** may correct cord compression.
- **Elevation of the presenting part** in the situation of a cord prolapse may minimize cord compression.
- **Amnioinfusion** can reestablish fluid volume in the uterus, thus, potentially creating a fluid cushion for the cord. This may also dilute meconium in an effort to prevent meconium aspiration.

Maximize Oxygenation

- Maternal position change
- Maternal supplemental oxygen
- Maternal breathing techniques
- Correct or treat underlying disease

28 © 2006 AWHONN

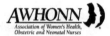

AWHONN
Association of Women's Health,
Obstetric and Neonatal Nurses

What are some ways we can maximize oxygenation of the fetus?

- **A lateral maternal position** that enhances utero-placental perfusion will maximize oxygen delivery to the fetus.
- With the application of **maternal supplemental oxygen,** we can maximize the oxygen delivery to the placenta by increasing maternal oxygen content.
- **Maternal breathing techniques** can be implemented to prevent hyperventilation and/or decrease maternal anxiety.
- **Correct or treat underlying disease. What are some examples of diseases that might affect maternal or fetal oxygenation?**

Anemia, cardiac structural defects, infection, pulmonary edema, hypertension.

Depending on the disease, the treatment may affect differing components of maternal or fetal oxygen transport. For example, treating infection will potentially decrease maternal and fetal oxygen consumption. Treatment for maternal anemia may improve ability of the mother's hemoglobin's to carry oxygen. Maternal or fetal transfusion of blood products may also increase maternal or fetal SaO_2. Treatment of a maternal respiratory disease may affect all components of maternal oxygen transport.

What component is targeted in the treatment of maternal hypertension?

Oxygen delivery to the tissues may improve with decreased vasoconstriction, allowing increased utero-placental blood flow.

Reduce Uterine Activity

- Maternal position change
- Reduce/discontinue uterotonic drugs
- Hydration
- Modified pushing
- Tocolytic medication

29 © 2006 AWHONN

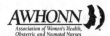

AWHONN
Association of Women's Health,
Obstetric and Neonatal Nurses

Our last goal addresses a reduction in uterine activity. Certainly, this goal would need to be addressed if the uterine activity is excessive. And, conversely, it would not be significant if the mother is not contracting. No matter what the uterine activity, it is necessary to assess the fetal tolerance to contractions. Even very minimal activity may not be tolerated by a fetus who may be compromised—this goal may even need to be addressed if the uterine activity is less than "adequate," as with commonly described parameters for "active labor."

Interventions to reduce uterine activity may include:

Maternal position change
Reduce/discontinue uterotonic drugs
Hydration
Modified pushing
Tocolytic medication

We have addressed all of these except the fourth one: modified pushing.

How can maternal pushing efforts be modified to address uterine activity?

Techniques such as delayed and nondirected pushing, open glottis pushing, and upright positioning can enhance maternal pushing efforts and/or fetal descent and decrease the time necessitated for maternal active pushing (AWHONN, 2000).

Be familiar with AWHONN's *Evidence-Based Clinical Practice Guideline: Nursing Management of the Second Stage of Labor.*

Assessment of Fetal Oxygenation and Acid-Base Status

Indirect methods:

- FHM
- Scalp stimulation
- Vibroacoustic stimulation
- Fetal movement assessment
- Fetal pulse oximetry

30 © 2006 AWHONN

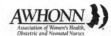

FHM is just one tool used to assess the maternal-fetal status. Traditionally, methods to assess fetal oxygenation have been achieved indirectly. These include those listed in this slide (Cypher & Adelsperger, 2003):

- **FHM**– including intermittent auscultation and palpation and electronic fetal monitoring
- **Scalp Stimulation**
- **Vibroacoustic stimulation**
  - These methods are based on agreement among experts that FHR accelerations usually indicate that a fetus is nonacidotic. **Fetal movement assessment** is based on the premise that the presence of fetal movement is a reassuring sign.
- **Fetal pulse oximetry** produces a real-time assessment of fetal oxygen saturation.

Assessment of Fetal Oxygenation and Acid-Base Status

Direct methods:

- Fetal scalp sampling
- Umbilical cord blood sampling

31 © 2006 AWHONN

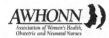

AWHONN
*Association of Women's Health,
Obstetric and Neonatal Nurses*

Direct methods of fetal oxygenation involve actual blood sampling. The two most commonly used methods are:

- **Fetal scalp sampling and**
- **Umbilical cord blood sampling.**

These two methods are discussed in length in the AWHONN FHMPP workshop, and, since you are experienced practitioners, our discussion here will be brief.

- Fetal scalp sampling is not presently utilized often in practice. It involves obtaining a sample of blood from the fetal scalp, testing its pH and watching the trend from multiple samples. Some reasons for its decline in use include its high cost, the difficulty in performing the procedure and the difficulty in obtaining a pure specimen.
- Umbilical cord blood sampling involves obtaining blood from the umbilical vessels and performing a blood gas analysis. Cord blood gas measurements provide an objective assessment of fetal status at delivery (Cypher & Adelsperger, 2003).
- A detailed description of these procedures and their interpretation is found in the AWHONN FHMPP textbook if you need more information.

Review Chapter 8 in the FHMPP textbook for further information.

AFMC Study Guide

Refer to the AWHONN *Fetal Heart Monitoring Principles and Practices* textbook for additional information

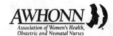

This concludes the review of information in the study guide. Additional information can be found in the AWHONN FHMPP textbook (specifically Chapters 2 and 3). To enhance your review and preparation for the AFMC additional information can also be obtained from the sources included in the reference list.

COURSE OUTLINE

AWHONN
Association of Women's Health,
Obstetric and Neonatal Nurses

Advanced Fetal Monitoring Course

©2006 AWHONN

Course Objectives

1. Identify basic physiologic principles underlying fetal heart monitoring.

2. Describe advanced physiologic principles of maternal and fetal oxygen transfer and acid-base balance.

3. Describe advanced concepts in antenatal testing including analysis & interpretation of biophysical profiles & complex antenatal fetal heart monitoring tracings.

4. Identify physiologic principles, goals & interventions for patients undergoing antenatal testing.

5. Evaluate the effectiveness of interventions for patients undergoing antenatal testing.

2 ©2006 AWHONN

Course Objectives (Cont.)

6. Compare and contrast physiologic principles and causes of adult cardiac dysrhythmias with fetal cardiac dysrhythmias.

7. Analyze fetal cardiac dysrhythmia patterns and describe outcomes associated with these patterns.

8. Analyze complex fetal heart monitoring patterns including uterine rupture, maternal-fetal hemorrhage, and abruption, utilizing National Institutes of Child Health and Human Development (NICHD) Fetal Heart Monitoring (FHR) nomenclature/definitions.

9. Apply perinatal risk management principles, communication techniques and documentation strategies related to complex and challenging patient care scenarios.

3 ©2006 AWHONN

Why Transition to NICHD?

- Standardization and simplification of key clinical terms and protocols are fundamental principles of patient safety

- Standardized terminology for fetal monitoring was recommended by Joint Commission on Accreditation of Healthcare Organizations (JCAHO) in the July 2004 Sentinel Event Alert #30

- Use of consistent FHM terminology among professional associations

4 ©2006 AWHONN

Potential Benefits

- Everyone on the perinatal team speaking the same language when communicating about fetal assessment data

- Clear, concise terms to minimize variation among care providers

- Consistency in medical record documentation of fetal status

- Decreased liability exposure

5 ©2006 AWHONN

Visual Determination of FHR Patterns

- NICHD definitions primarily were developed for visual interpretation

- Mathematical quantification of definitions are general guidelines

- Quantitative and qualitative interpretation

- "In most cases"; "approximate" included in definitions

6 ©2006 AWHONN

Visual Determination (Cont.)

- Definitions apply to interpretation of FHR patterns produced from either a direct fetal electrode detecting the fetal electrocardiogram or an external Doppler device detecting the fetal heart events with use of the autocorrelation technique.

- Assuming a readable tracing is obtained, there is no inherent need for amniotomy, spiral electrode and/or intrauterine pressure catheter insertion for FHR pattern interpretation.

7 ©2006 AWHONN

Determination and Documentation of Baseline Rate

- Baseline rate is the approximate mean FHR rounded to increments of 5 bpm during a 10 minute segment, excluding:
  - ➢ Periodic or episodic (previously known as nonperiodic) changes
  - ➢ Periods of marked FHR variability
  - ➢ Segments of the baseline that differ by >25 bpm
- Baseline rate can be determined between contractions
- Rate plus baseline variability gives the indication of range (for example, 135 bpm with moderate variability implies a range of 6 to 25 bpm)

8 ©2006 AWHONN

Determination and Documentation of Baseline Rate (Cont.)

- In any 10 minute window, the minimum baseline duration must be at least 2 minutes or the baseline for that period is indeterminate.

- In this case, one may need to refer to the previous 10 minute segment(s) for determination of the baseline.

9 ©2006 AWHONN

Periodic and Episodic Patterns

- Accelerations and decelerations are categorized as either periodic or episodic.
- Periodic patterns are those associated with uterine contractions.
- Episodic patterns are those not associated with uterine contractions (formerly known as *nonperiodic*).

10 ©2006 AWHONN

Baseline Variability

- No distinction is made between short-term variability (or beat-to-beat variability or R-R wave period differences in the ECG) and long-term variability because in actual practice they are visually determined as a unit.

- Hence the definition of variability is based on visual assessment of the amplitude of the complexes, with exclusion of the regular, smooth sinusoidal pattern.

11 ©2006 AWHONN

Variability – NICHD Terminology

Amplitude of FHR Change	Former AWHONN Baseline LTV Description	NICHD Baseline Variability Description
Undetectable from baseline	Decreased/Minimal	Absent
Visually detectable from baseline, ≤ 5 bpm	Decreased/Minimal	Minimal
6 – 25 bpm	Average/Within Normal Limits	Moderate
> 25 bpm	Marked/Saltatory	Marked

12 | ©2006 AWHONN

NICHD Baseline Variability

Undetectable from baseline Absent	
Visually detectable from baseline, ≤ 5 bpm Minimal	
6 – 25 bpm Moderate	
>25 bpm Marked	

13 ©2006 AWHONN

Accelerations

Visually apparent abrupt increase from FHR baseline
Term: ▪ Onset to peak < 30 seconds; acme ≥ 15 bpm ▪ Duration ≥ 15 seconds < 2 minutes
Preterm: ▪ Onset to peak < 30 seconds acme ≥ 10 bpm ▪ Duration ≥10 seconds
Prolonged acceleration duration ≥ 2 minutes < 10 minutes

14 ©2006 AWHONN

Early Decelerations

Visually apparent gradual decrease and return to FHR baseline associated with uterine contraction
Onset to nadir ≥ 30 seconds
Nadir occurs at peak of contraction

15 ©2006 AWHONN

Late Decelerations

Visually apparent gradual decrease and return to baseline FHR associated with contractions
Onset to nadir $\geq$ 30 seconds
Onset, nadir, and recovery occur after onset, peak and recovery of contraction

16 ©2006 AWHONN

Variable Decelerations

Visually apparent abrupt decrease from FHR baseline; may occur with or without contractions
Onset to beginning of nadir < 30 seconds
Decrease $\geq$ 15 bpm Duration $\geq$ 15 seconds and < 2 minutes from onset to return to baseline FHR

17 ©2006 AWHONN

Variable Decelerations (Cont.)

- Variable decelerations inherently vary in timing, shape and duration.

- They should be described as variable decelerations *without* additional clarification of atypical features

18 ©2006 AWHONN

Prolonged Decelerations

Visually apparent decrease in FHR below baseline

Decrease $\geq$ 15 bpm
Duration $\geq$ 2 minutes and < 10 minutes from onset to return to baseline

19 ©2006 AWHONN

Combination Decelerations

- Not all FHR patterns will meet the mathematical criteria in the NICHD definitions exactly.
- Choose the *one* definition that most closely approximates the FHR pattern displayed.
- Terms such as "early variable decelerations," "late variable decelerations," "variable decelerations with a late component," or "variable in shape, but late in timing" are inconsistent with NICHD definitions.
- Some 10 minute segments may have two or more types of decelerations; identify each type of deceleration appropriately.

20 ©2006 AWHONN

More than one type of deceleration within a 10 minute segment

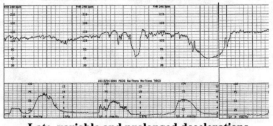

Late, variable and prolonged decelerations

21 ©2006 AWHONN

Persistent vs. Recurrent

- Decelerations are defined as *recurrent* if they occur with ≥50% of uterine contractions in any 20 minute segment.

- The term *persistent* has been used in the past to describe repetitive FHR patterns but has not been precisely defined.

- In some cases, persistency has been defined as *usually* occurring with ≥50% of contractions without a time frame (e.g. 20 minute segment).

22 ©2006 AWHONN

Systematic Assessment of FHR Tracings

- Baseline rate
- Variability
- Periodic/episodic changes
- Uterine Activity
- Pattern evolution
- Accompanying clinical characteristics
- Urgency

Adapted from Fox, Kilpatrick, King & Parer, (2000)

23 ©2006 AWHONN

Definitions of Key Terms

- Acidemia: ↑concentration of hydrogen ions in the blood
- Acidosis: ↑ concentration of hydrogen ions in the tissue
- Hypoxemia: ↓ oxygen content in the blood
- Hypoxia: ↓ level of oxygen in the tissue
- Asphyxia: damaging hypoxia, acidemia and metabolic acidosis

(ACOG, 2003; ACOG, 1995)

24 ©2006 AWHONN

Oxygenated Term Fetus

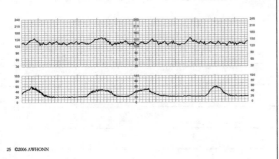

25 ©2006 AWHONN

Neonatal Encephalopathy and Cerebral Palsy

Four criteria to define an acute intrapartum event sufficient to cause cerebral palsy (ACOG, 2003 p. xviii):

- Evidence of metabolic acidosis in fetal umbilical arterial blood obtained at delivery (pH <7 and base deficit ≥12 mmol/L)

26 ©2006 AWHONN

Neonatal Encephalopathy and Cerebral Palsy (Cont.)

Criteria continued:

- Early onset of severe or moderate neonatal encephalopathy in infants born at 34 or more weeks of gestation

(ACOG, 2003)

27 ©2006 AWHONN

Neonatal Encephalopathy and Cerebral Palsy (Cont.)

Neonatal Encephalopathy:

- "A clinically defined syndrome of disturbed neurologic function in the earliest days of life in the term infant, manifested by difficulty with initiating and maintaining respiration, depression of tone and reflexes, subnormal level of consciousness, and often by seizures"

(ACOG, 2003, p.84)

28 ©2006 AWHONN

Neonatal Encephalopathy and Cerebral Palsy (Cont.)

Criteria continued:

- Cerebral palsy of spastic quadriplegic or dyskinetic type

(ACOG, 2003)

29 ©2006 AWHONN

Types of Cerebral Palsy (CP)

Spastic	Athetoid/Dyskinetic
- 70-80% of individuals with CP - Characterized by stiff muscles - Spastic quadriplegia most severe form & associated with mental retardation	- 10-20% of individuals with CP - Characterized by fluctuations in muscle tone, uncontrolled movement - Associated with sucking, swallowing, speech impediments

30 ©2006 AWHONN

Neonatal Encephalopathy and Cerebral Palsy (Cont.)

Criteria continued:

- Exclusion of other identifiable etiologies such as trauma, coagulation disorders, infectious conditions, or genetic disorders

(ACOG, 2003)

31   ©2006 AWHONN

Oxygen Transport

Four components of oxygen transport:
- Oxygen content — what's in blood — plasma + hemoglobin
- Oxygen affinity — PaO_2 — how well it sticks to hemoglobin [SaO₂]
- Oxygen delivery
- Oxygen consumption

(Harvey & Chez, 1997)

32   ©2006 AWHONN

full sat. hemoglobin molecule can carry 4 O2 molecule

Maternal Oxygen Transport

Maternal oxygen content:

- The total amount of oxygen in the maternal arterial blood
- Components:
  - Amount of oxygen dissolved in plasma (PaO_2)
  - Percent of oxygen carried on the hemoglobin (SaO_2)

33   ©2006 AWHONN

Maternal Oxygen Transport (Cont.)

- PaO_2 helps bind O_2 molecules to hemoglobin
- Saturated hemoglobin molecule carries four molecules of O_2
- SaO_2 more precise measure of oxygen content than PaO_2

34 ©2006 AWHONN

Maternal Oxygen Transport (Cont.)

Oxygen affinity:

- The reversible binding and unbinding of oxygen to hemoglobin
- Can change with variations in pH, CO_2, maternal temperature

35 ©2006 AWHONN

Maternal Oxyhemoglobin Dissociation Curve

36 ©2006 AWHONN

Maternal Oxygen Transport (Cont.)

Oxygen delivery:

- Amount of oxygen delivered to the tissues each minute
- Two components are:
  - Oxygen content
  - Cardiac output

37 ©2006 AWHONN

Maternal Oxygen Transport (Cont.)

Oxygen consumption:

Amount of oxygen consumed by the body and tissues each minute

38 ©2006 AWHONN

Fetal Oxygen Transport

- Includes O_2 content, affinity, delivery, and consumption
- Is directly dependent on maternal O_2 transport
- Is affected by:
  - Blood flow to the uterus and placenta
  - Integrity of the placenta
  - Blood flow through the umbilical cord

39 ©2006 AWHONN

Fetal Oxygen Transport (Cont.)

Fetal oxygen content:

- Amount of oxygen dissolved in plasma (PaO_2)
- Amount of oxygen carried on the hemoglobin (SaO_2)

40 ©2006 AWHONN

Fetal Oxygen Transport (Cont.)

- Fetal oxygen tension is about 25% that of an adult
- Fetal hemoglobin:
  - Has an increased oxygen affinity
  - Has a higher concentration than maternal (approximately 17 gm/dl at term)

(Freeman, 2003; Harvey & Chez, 1997)

41 ©2006 AWHONN

Fetal Oxygen Transport (Cont.)

42 ©2006 AWHONN

Fetal Oxygen Transport (Cont.)

Oxygen delivery:

Fetal O_2 delivery system facilitates optimal fetal oxygenation and growth through unique circulation patterns.

43 ©2006 AWHONN

Fetal Circulation

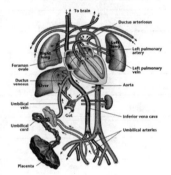

44 ©2006 AWHONN

Fetal Oxygen Transport (Cont.)

■ Fetal oxygen consumption:
  ➢ Fetus attempts to decrease O_2 consumption if needs not met
■ Altered fetal O_2 consumption may result in:
  ➢ Changes in the FHR
  ➢ ↓ fetal movement
  ➢ Alterations in behavioral state
  ➢ Fetal growth deceleration
  ➢ ↓ fetal tissue perfusion

45 ©2006 AWHONN

JoAnn, 17 Years Old
G1 P0, 40 $^5/_7$ Weeks' Gestation

- Family history: None provided
- Medical history:
  - Car accident, broken arm and facial laceration
- Previous pregnancies: denies
- Psychosocial history:
  - In an abusive relationship
  - Not in school
  - Not living with parents

46 ©2006 AWHONN

JoAnn (Cont.)
Current Pregnancy

- Four prenatal visits; two different providers
- First trimester substance abuse
- Current tobacco use
- Normal prenatal lab values

47 ©2006 AWHONN

JoAnn (Cont.)
Admission Data

- Spontaneous uterine contractions, q 5-6 min
- SROM 0655:
  - Grossly ruptured membranes
  - Fern positive; clear fluid; no odor
- SVE: 1-2/80%/-1; vertex presentation
- VS: BP 119/73, P 75, R 20, afebrile

48 ©2006 AWHONN

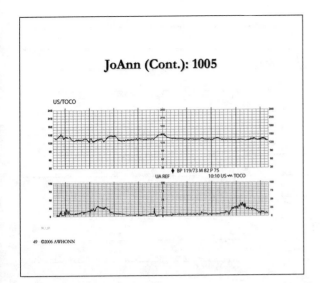

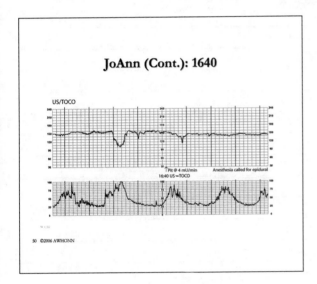

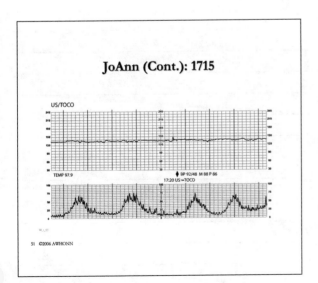

Effects of Ephedrine

- Maternal
  - ➢ ↑ Heart rate
  - ➢ ↑ Cardiac output
  - ➢ ↑ Blood pressure
- Fetal
  - ➢ ↑ baseline FHR
  - ➢ Tachycardia
  - ➢ ↑ FHR variability, accelerations

52 ©2006 AWHONN

JoAnn (Cont.): 1800

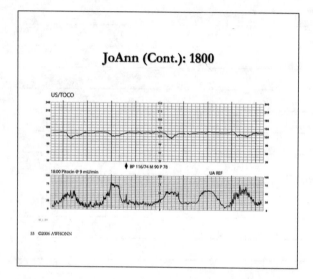

53 ©2006 AWHONN

JoAnn (Cont.): 1925

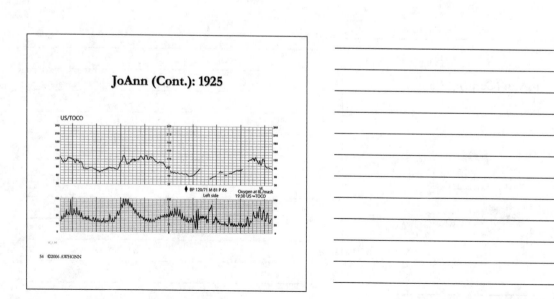

54 ©2006 AWHONN

Beta adrenergic

doesn't shunt from
uterus

Sudafed +

JoAnn (Cont.): 1938

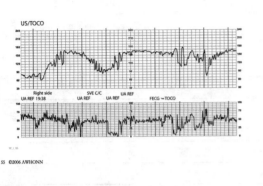

JoAnn (Cont.)
Outcome

- Cesarean birth with epidural anesthesia
- Male infant: 6 lb, 7 oz; (2920 grams)
- Apgar scores: 1/6/7
- Moderate clot in uterine cavity, partial abruption
- Nuchal cord X2; very thin cord
- Grade III placenta with calcification

FHM in the Preterm Fetus

- The preterm fetus's physiologic responses are dependent on the stage of fetal development
- The preterm fetus's physiologic responses and tolerance to stress can differ from those in the term fetus

Preterm FHR Characteristics

- The FHR baseline may be higher
- Accelerations may be of lower amplitude
- Variability may be decreased
- Variable decelerations occur more frequently

58 ©2006 AWHONN

FHM in the Preterm Fetus

- Magnesium sulfate may affect the FHR by decreasing the FHR variability
- Beta-sympathomimetics, such as terbutaline, frequently cause tachycardia in both the mother and fetus
- Antenatal steroids may affect FHR variability

59 ©2006 AWHONN

Sympathetic — speedy
Parasympathetic — pokey

Intrapartum Preterm FHR Pattern Characteristics

- Variable decelerations occur more frequently
- Tachycardia and decreased variability occur more frequently
- Late and prolonged decelerations occur at the same frequency as term fetus

60 ©2006 AWHONN

70-78% of laboring preterm infant

Preterm Fetal Tolerance to Stress

- The preterm fetus is more likely to be subjected to hypoxia
- Preterm FHR patterns progress more rapidly from reassuring to nonreassuring than at term
- Variable decelerations and tachycardia with loss of variability are associated with acidosis and low Apgar scores in the preterm fetus

(Freeman et al., 2003)

61 ©2006 AWHONN

Maya, 28 Years Old
G1 P0, 27 $^4/_7$ Weeks Gestation, PPROM

- Family history: Mother has hypertension
- Medical history: Appendectomy, age 15
- Previous pregnancies: Denies
- Psychosocial history:
  - ➤ Dropped out of high school
  - ➤ Married, good support network
- Leaking clear amniotic fluid on admission

62 ©2006 AWHONN

Maya (Cont.) NST Day Five

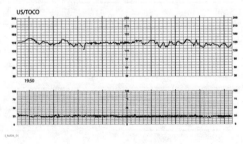

63 ©2006 AWHONN

Maya (Cont.): 22 Hours Later, 1732

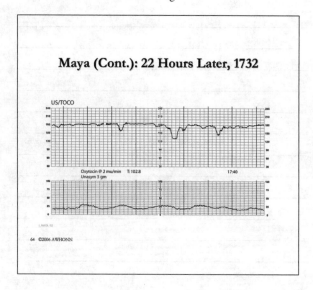

US/TOCO

Oxytocin @ 2 mu/min   T: 102.8   17:40
Unasym 3 gm

64 ©2006 AWHONN

Maya (Cont.): 1750

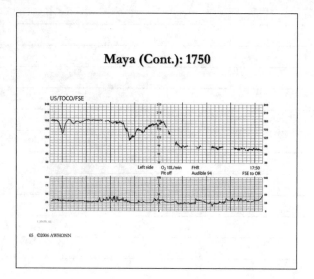

US/TOCO/FSE

Left side   O₂ 10L/min   FHR   17:50
            Pit off   Audible 94   FSE to OR

65 ©2006 AWHONN

The Physiologic Basis for Advanced Fetal Heart Monitoring

- Physiologic principles underlying fetal heart monitoring
- Advanced physiologic principles of maternal and fetal oxygen transfer and acid-base balance
- The nursing process and its relationship to fetal heart monitoring

66 ©2006 AWHONN

Antepartum Fetal Assessment

67 ©2006 AWHONN

Indications for Antepartum Testing

- Decreased uteroplacental blood flow
- Decreased gas exchange
- Abnormal metabolic processes
- Fetal sepsis
- Fetal anemia
- Fetal heart rate failure
- Umbilical cord accident candidates

68 ©2006 AWHONN   (Kontopoulos & Vintzileos, 2004)

**Examples of
Maternal-Fetal Conditions**

- Hypertension
- Postdates pregnancy
- Fetal hyperglycemia
- Preterm premature rupture of membranes
- Fetomaternal hemorrhage
- Cardiac arrhythmia
- Umbilical cord entanglement

69 ©2006 AWHONN

Fetal Response to Hypoxemia

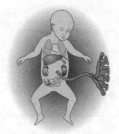 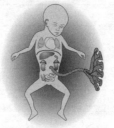

Normoxia   Hypoxia

70 ©2006 AWHONN

Methods of Antepartum Fetal Testing

- Fetal Movement Counts (FMC)
- Nonstress Test (NST)
- Vibroacoustic Stimulation (VAS)
- Contraction Stress Test (CST)
- Oxytocin Challenge Test (OCT)
- Biophysical Profile (BPP)
- Modified Biophysical Profile
- Doppler Flow Studies

71 ©2006 AWHONN

Fetal Movement Counts (FMC)

- Perception of fetal movement by the woman
- Important assessment of fetal health
- Variety of FMC methods, ideal number of movements and optimal counting duration not defined

72 ©2006 AWHONN

Example of FMC Method

- Select consistent time of day
- Count fetal movement during a specified period
- Chart time the 10th movement felt
- Call provider for:
  - < 10 movements
  - Longer period required to achieve 10 movements than on previous days

Factors Influencing Fetal Movement

- Time of day
- Tobacco ↓ FM for up to 80 mins
- Medications (narcotics)
- Maternal physical activity
- Maternal anxiety

Nonstress Test

- Primary antepartum assessment tool
- External assessment of:
  - Fetal heart rate
  - Oxygenation
  - Neurologic function
  - Cardiac function

Physiology of Antepartum Testing

- Acceleration of the heart rate in response to fetal movement
- Accelerations, fetal movement and variability usually exclude acidemia

76 ©2006 AWHONN

NST Interpretation

- Reactive
  - Two or more FHR accelerations ≥15 bpm above baseline, lasting ≥15 seconds within 20 minutes
- Nonreactive
  - No FHR accelerations meeting criteria within a maximum of 40 minutes

77 ©2006 AWHONN

Preterm Fetus <32 Weeks of Gestation and NST Interpretation

- Reactive
  - Two or more FHR accelerations ≥10 bpm above baseline, lasting ≥10 seconds within 20 minutes (may be extended to 60-90 minutes)
- Nonreactive
  - No FHR accelerations meeting criteria within a maximum of 90 minutes

78 ©2006 AWHONN

Reactive NST

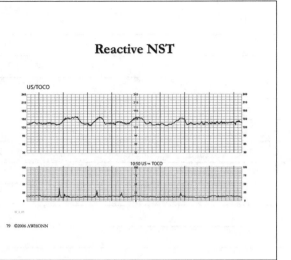

US/TOCO

10:50 US → TOCO

79 ©2006 AWHONN

Nonreactive NST

US/TOCO

11:30 US → TOCO

80 ©2006 AWHONN

Variable Decelerations and NST

- Variable decelerations may occur during the NST
- Nonrepetitive lasting <30 seconds
- Repetitive (3 or more in 20 minutes)

81 ©2006 AWHONN

Vibroacoustic Stimulation (VAS)

- Evaluation of FHR response to acoustic stimulation
  - ➤ Establish baseline
  - ➤ Apply up to 3-second stimulus near fetal head
  - ➤ May repeat every 1 minute up to three times
- Two or more accelerations in a 20-minute period after stimulus

82 ©2006 AWHONN

VAS (Cont.)

US/TOCO

↓ VAS
20:30 US ≈ TOCO

83 ©2006 AWHONN

Contraction Stress Test
Oxytocin Challenge Test

CST	OCT
Endogenous oxytocin	Exogenous oxytocin
Breast/nipple stimulation	IV infusion pump
Response to ↓ O_2 during contractions	Response to ↓ O_2 during contractions

84 ©2006 AWHONN

Indications and Contraindications

- Indications
  - Nonreactive NST
- Contraindications
  - Preterm premature rupture of membranes
  - Placenta previa
  - Prior classical incision or uterine surgery
  - Preterm labor

Test Procedure

- Semi-fowlers or lateral position
- Baseline maternal vital signs
- FHR and uterine activity monitoring
- IV oxytocin or nipple stimulation
- Goal:
  - Observe three or more contractions lasting 40 seconds each in a 10-minute period

Negative OCT

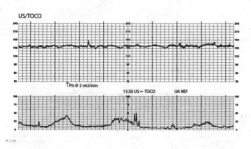

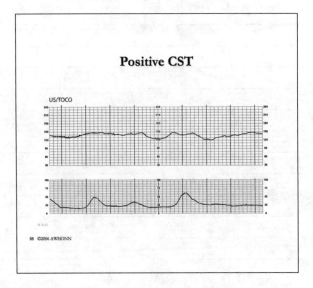

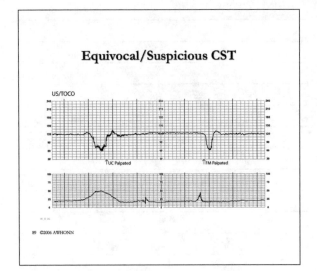

Intermittent lates
or variables

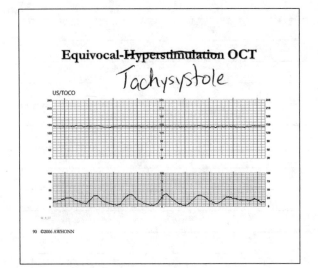

Tachysystole –
25 ctx in 10 mins

Unsatisfactory CST

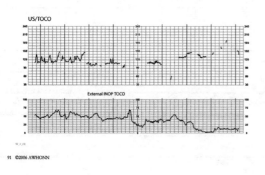

91 ©2006 AWHONN

Biophysical Profile (BPP) Interpretation

- Combination of NST and four ultrasound biophysical characteristics:
  - Fetal movement
  - Fetal tone
  - Fetal breathing
  - Amniotic fluid volume
- Score of 0 or 2 points for each parameter

92 ©2006 AWHONN

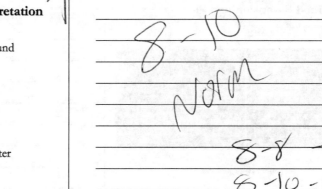

BPP Interpretation

Parameter	Normal (2)	Abnormal (0)
Reactive FHR	At least two episodes FHR acceleration of 15x15 with FM in 30 min	< 2 episodes of acceleration of FHR or acceleration <15 bpm in 30 minutes
Fetal breathing	At least 1 episode fetal breathing movement (FBM) of at least 30 sec within 30 minutes	Absent FBM or no episode of ≥30 seconds in 30 minutes
Gross body movement	At least 3 discrete body/limb movements in 30 minutes (active continuous movement episode equals a single movement)	≤ 2 episodes of body/limb movements in 30 minutes

93 ©2006 AWHONN

BPP Interpretation (Cont.)

Parameter	Normal (2)	Abnormal (0)
Fetal tone	At least 1 episode active extension with return to flexion of fetal limbs or trunk. Opening and closing of hand equals normal tone	Slow extension, return to partial flexion; or movement of limb in full extension; or absent FM With fetal hand in complete or partial deflection
Qualitative AFV	At least 1 pocket of amniotic fluid (AF) that measures at least 2 cm in 2 perpendicular planes	No AF pockets; or pocket < 2 cm in two perpendicular planes

94 ©2006 AWHONN

Hand Extension and Flexion

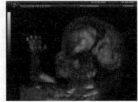 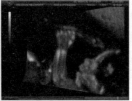

Images used with permission of GE Healthcare

95 ©2006 AWHONN

Interpretation and Suggested Management for BPP

Considerations:

- Maternal-fetal status
- Bishop score
- Gestational age
- Fetal lung maturity status
- Other pertinent history or physical assessment data

96 ©2006 AWHONN

Modified BPP

NST and Amniotic Fluid Index (AFI)

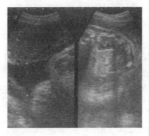

- Largest vertical pocket in four quadrants
- AFI = total of four quadrants

Image used with permission of The Institute for Advanced Medical Education

97 ©2006 AWHONN

Doppler Flow Studies

- Ultrasound using Doppler technology
- Measures blood flow within arteries:
  - ➢ Uterine artery
  - ➢ Umbilical artery
  - ➢ Middle cerebral artery
- Rising systolic/diastolic ratios = ↓ blood flow to the placenta

98 ©2006 AWHONN

Interpretation

- Normal flow

- Absent end diastolic flow

- Reverse end diastolic flow

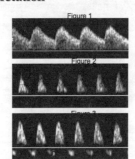

Figure 1

Figure 2

Figure 3

99 ©2006 AWHONN   Images used with permission of GE Healthcare

Margaret, 30 years old
G_2P_{1001}, 32 $^2/_7$ weeks

- Family History-unremarkable
- Medical/Surgical History-unremarkable
- Pregnancy History:
  - SVD at 37 weeks for preeclampsia
  - PUPPS during third trimester
  - Viable male infant, 6 lbs 13 oz
- Current Pregnancy
  - Abnormal triple marker screening test
  - Normal Level II ultrasound, declined amniocentesis

100 ©2006 AWHONN

Margaret: Admission Tracing

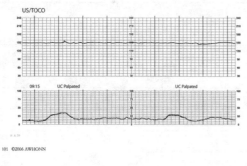

101 ©2006 AWHONN

Margaret: 0920

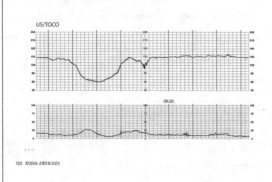

102 ©2006 AWHONN

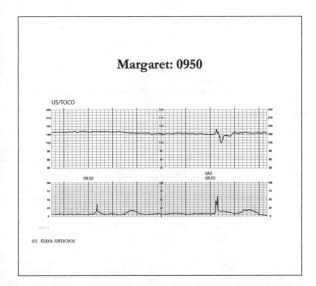

Margaret: 0950

103 ©2006 AWHONN

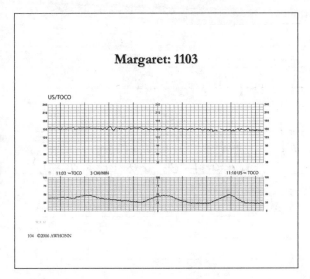

Margaret: 1103

104 ©2006 AWHONN

Margaret's Outcome

■ Delivered at 1152

■ Viable female infant:

➤ Apgars 2/6/7

➤ Cystic formations on umbilical cord

➤ No signs of placental abruption

105 ©2006 AWHONN

Summary

- Antepartum fetal testing is a valuable and important component of prenatal care, particularly for at-risk women

- Goal is to identify techniques that are user friendly and minimally invasive and yield the most useful information

106 ©2006 AWHONN

Why Study Fetal Dysrhythmias and Arrhythmias?

- Fetal dysrhythmias and arrhythmias can:
  - Affect fetal cardiac output, FHR & pattern
  - Make tracing interpretation challenging
- Knowledge can facilitate assessment, patient, and family education

107 ©2006 AWHONN

Definition of Terms

Terms	Examples
Dysrhythmia: Abnormal FHR due to abnormalities in the P-QRS relationship	Early P waves Wide or bizarre-looking QRS complexes **Examples:** Atrial flutter and complete heart block
Arrhythmia: FHR without rhythm	Sporadic, irregular beats associated with variation in R-R interval with normal P waves **Example:** Marked variability

108 ©2006 AWHONN

Arrhythmia

A — no rhythm
(marked variability)

D

Cardiac and Conduction System Development

Gestation (Weeks)	Developmental Milestones
3	Tubular heart beating
4	Tube folds; atrial and ventricular septa forming SA node developing
5	Atrial and ventricular septa AV node & bundle of His developing
6	Valves forming Coronary circulation established

109 ©2006 AWHONN

Comparison of Cardiac Characteristics

Factor	Fetus	Adult
Contractile mass	30%	60%
Calcium Transport	Altered	Fully functional
Cardiac Pressures	High on right side (atrium)	High on left side
Cardiac output (CO)	RV output + LV output	LV output

110 ©2006 AWHONN

Cardiac Conduction Physiology

111 ©2006 AWHONN

Properties of Cardiac Cells

- Automaticity:
  - ➢ Ability to spontaneously contract without neural stimulation
- Excitability:
  - ➢ Ability to respond to electrical stimulus
- Conductivity:
  - ➢ Ability to conduct electrical impulses through cardiac cells

112 ©2006 AWHONN

Cardiac Conduction System

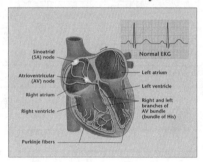

113 ©2006 AWHONN

ECG pattern

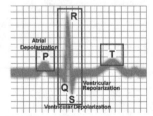

114 ©2006 AWHONN

Etiology of Dysrhythmias

- Congenital heart defects
  - SVT
  - Atrial flutter
  - Complete heart block
- Conduction system defects
- Cardiomyopathies
  - Infant of diabetic mother
  - Twin-to-twin transfusion

115 ©2006 AWHONN

Etiology of Dysrhythmias (Cont.)

- Disease processes such as:
  - Systemic lupus erythematosus (SLE)
- Viral infections:
  - Cytomegalovirus *herpes family*
  - Rubella
  - Parvovirus

116 ©2006 AWHONN

Sinus Node Variants: Tachycardia

117 ©2006 AWHONN

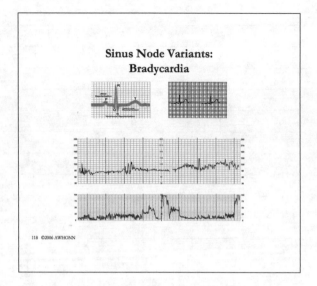

Sinus Node Variants:
Bradycardia

118 ©2006 AWHONN

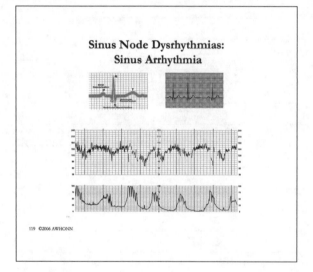

Sinus Node Dysrhythmias:
Sinus Arrhythmia

119 ©2006 AWHONN

Mary, 34 year old
$G_1 P_{0,}$ **41 weeks gestation**

- Family history: negative
- Medical/Surgical history: negative
- Married and has support
- Pregnancy has been uncomplicated
- Spontaneous rupture of membranes (SROM), clear fluid, 12 hr. before admission
- Fetal movement present
- Mild, irregular uterine contractions

120 ©2006 AWHONN

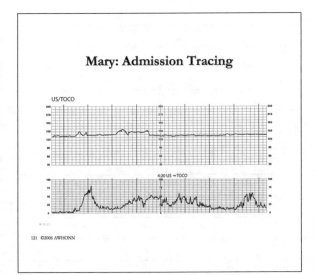

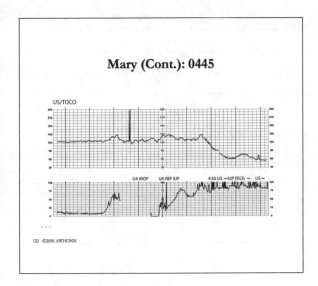

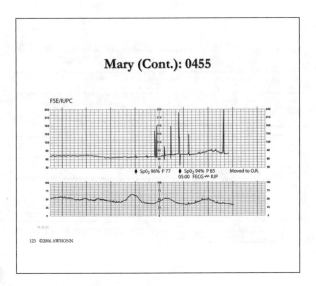

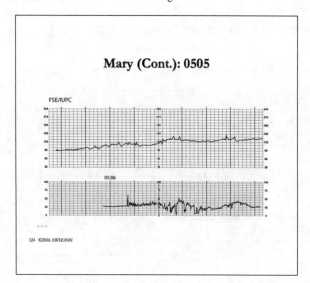

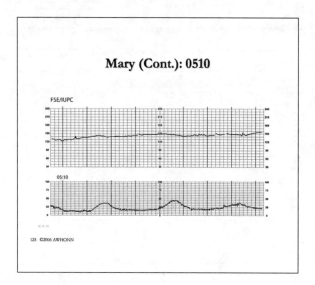

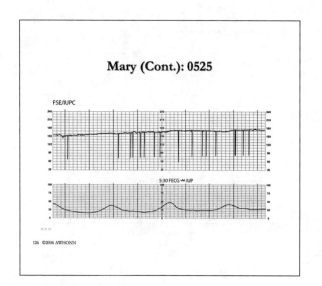

Mary (Cont.): 1035
5 Hours Since Last Tracing

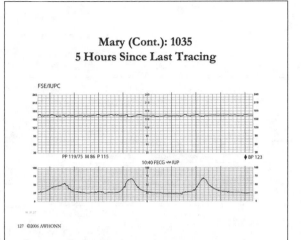

Atrial Dysrhythmias:
Premature Atrial Contractions (PACs)

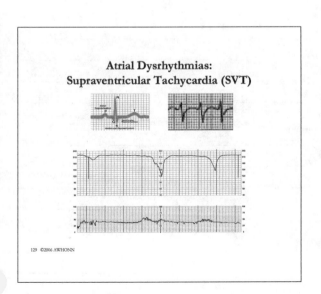

caffien, nicotine, stress

Atrial Dysrhythmias:
Supraventricular Tachycardia (SVT)

Esperanza, 25 years old
G_1 P_0, 24 weeks of gestation

- Family history: negative
- Medical/surgical history: negative
- Current pregnancy:
  - First prenatal visit
- Psychosocial history:
  - Unmarried
  - Migrant worker
  - Does not speak English

130 ©2006 AWHONN

Esperanza: (Cont.)
Assessment Process

- Auscultated FHR >200 bpm x 2
- Referred to a tertiary center:
  - Fetal echocardiogram
  - Ultrasound
- Gestational age now 24 $^5/_7$ weeks

131 ©2006 AWHONN

Esperanza: (Cont.)
Echocardiogram and Ultrasound

- No structural cardiac abnormalities
- Fetal hydrops: CHF   CHF
  - Abdominal fluid present
  - Scalp edema present

132 ©2006 AWHONN

Esperanza: (Cont.)
Treatment Plan

- Admitted to Labor and Delivery
- Digoxin therapy planned to convert rhythm
- Continuous fetal heart monitoring initiated
- Plan for continued medical and nursing care and evaluation of therapy explained

133 ©2006 AWHONN

Esperanza: (Cont.)
Admission Findings

- 25 weeks gestation
- Vital signs:
  - 110/70, 72, 22, 97.5°F (36.4°C)
- Baseline FHR 120 via external ultrasound
- No uterine contractions, vaginal bleeding, or leaking of amniotic fluid
- Fetal movement present

134 ©2006 AWHONN

Esperanza: (Cont.)

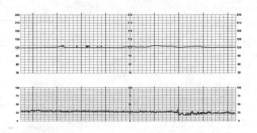

135 ©2006 AWHONN

Esperanza: (Cont.)

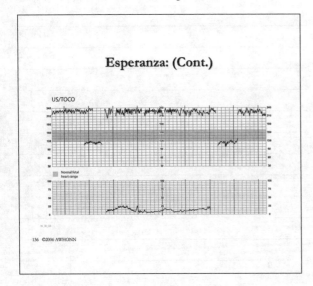

Esperanza: (Cont.)
Outcome

- Fetus converted to sinus rhythm within five days
- Digoxin continued on outpatient basis, then tapered off
- Delivered baby girl at 39 weeks:
  - ➤ 7 lbs., 8 oz. (3402 grams)
  - ➤ Apgars 9 and 9 at 1 and 5 minutes

Atrial Dysrhythmias: (Cont.)
Atrial Flutter

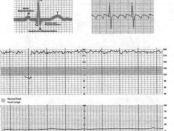

Junctional and Ventricular Dysrhythmias: AV Node Blocks

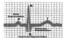

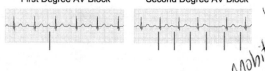

First Degree AV Block   Second Degree AV Block

139 ©2006 AWHONN

widens P-Q interval until dropped beat

Mobitz 1
Mobitz 2

Junctional and Ventricular Dysrhythmias: Third Degree AV Node Block

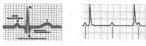

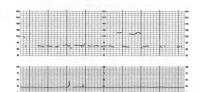

140 ©2006 AWHONN

SSA ⟋ antibodies
SSB
lupus
rheumatoid arthritis

Junctional and Ventricular Dysrhythmias Premature Ventricular Contractions (PVCs)

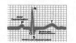
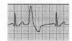

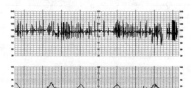

141 ©2006 AWHONN

myocarditis
hyperkalemia

Potential Consequences of Fetal Dysrhythmias

Potential continuum of consequences:

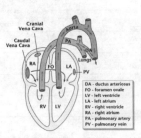

- No apparent effect
- Fetal hydrops
- Death

DA - ductus arteriosus
FO - foramen ovale
LV - left ventricle
LA - left atrium
RV - right ventricle
RA - right atrium
PA - pulmonary artery
PV - pulmonary vein

142 ©2006 AWHONN

Diagnosing Dysrhythmias

- Spectral Doppler and color flow mapping
- Fetal echocardiography
- M-mode echocardiography

143 ©2006 AWHONN

Treatment of Dysrhythmias

PACs, PVCs	Avoid caffeine, sympathomimetic medications
Atrial Flutter SVT	Administer digoxin Consider other antiarrhythmic medications
AV Block	Consider sympathomometic medications, betamethasone
Consider delivery for worsening fetal condition regardless of gestational age or deliver at term if stable	

144 ©2006 AWHONN

Dysrhythmia Section Conclusion

- Incidence is rare
- Diagnostic and follow-up testing during prenatal period
- Assessment of impact of ↓ fetal cardiac output on well-being
- Treatment plan based on specific dysrhythmia
- Variable outcomes

145 ©2006 AWHONN

Complex Case Scenarios and Their Related Maternal - Fetal Physiology

- Focus on overall picture - nursing process
- Assessment - History, physical exam, psychosocial issues
- Interpretation - FHR and uterine activity
- Diagnosis - What is the risk?
- Intervention - Actions (physiologic goals)
- Evaluation - Communication & documentation

146 ©2006 AWHONN

Sally, 20 Years Old
G2 P$_{0101}$ 35 Weeks Gestation

- Family History:
  - Mother – hypertension
  - Both parents – congestive heart failure (CHF)
  - Maternal Grandmother – Type 2 diabetes
- Medical History:
  - Chlamydia 4 years prior to pregnancy
  - Smokes ½ pack/day
  - Allergic to penicillin
  - Previous surgery: wisdom teeth extraction

147 ©2006 AWHONN

Sally: (Cont.)
Current Pregnancy

Gestation	Symptoms	BP/FHR
35 weeks	C/O faintness, nausea, spots before eyes No edema	BP 136/96 FHR 159 bpm
37 weeks	2 to 3+ patellar reflexes 2+ pitting edema	BP range: 138/84 to 153/114 Reactive NST

148 ©2006 AWHONN

Sally:(Cont.)
Three Days Later

Gestation	Symptoms	BP/FHR
$37^3/_7$ weeks	Headache, 2+ proteinuria, 1+ bilateral patellar reflexes	BP range: 136/102 to 133/83 FHR 155 bpm

Noncompliant with bed rest at home

149 ©2006 AWHONN

Blood Pressure Measurement

- Measure BP in same arm, same position whenever possible
  - BP cuff at heart level
- Sitting, standing position:
  - Systolic BP (SBP) → Minimal change through pregnancy
  - Diastolic BP (DBP) → Decreases through first and second trimester, increases toward term
- Left lateral recumbent position:
  - SBP and DBP → Decrease through second trimester, increase toward term

150 ©2006 AWHONN

BP Measurement (Cont.)

- Auscultate diastolic BP as disappearance of sound (Korotkoff phase V)
- Choose correct cuff size
  - ➢ Encircles ≥80% arm circumference
- Use same device whenever possible

151 ©2006 AWHONN

Sally: (Cont.)
Admission Data

- Admitted at 2232 for bright red bleeding, leaking fluid and abdominal pain
- VS:
  - ➢ BP 183/105, P 130, R 24, T 98.9° F (37.1° C)
- Patellar reflexes: 3+; 0 clonus
- VE: 3 cm/90%/+1; anterior/soft cervix
- Unable to void

152 ©2006 AWHONN

Sally:(Cont.)
Laboratory Values

HELLP (handwritten)

WBC:	15.23 x 10⁹/L (10^9)	Fibrinogen:	300 mg/dL
RBC:	3.54 x 10¹²/L (10^{12})	Uric Acid:	7.1 mg/dL ↑
Hct:	30.7%	Alk Phos:	253 IU/ml
Hgb:	11.0 g/dL	AST:	15 IU
↓ Platelets:	141K/mm³	ALT:	14 IU
PT:	9.9 secs	LDH:	542 IU ↑
PTT:	30 secs	Urine drug screen neg	

creatinine (handwritten)

153 ©2006 AWHONN

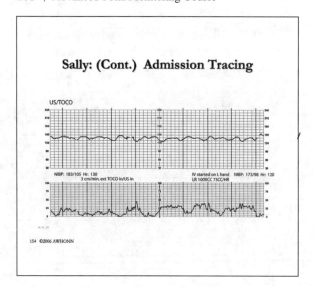

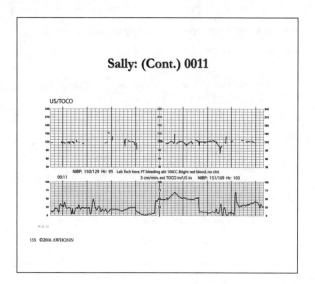

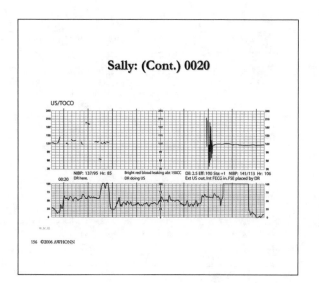

Sally: (Cont) 0029

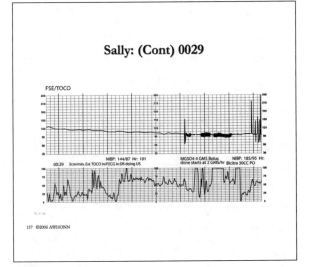

Sally: (Cont.) 0048 (OR)

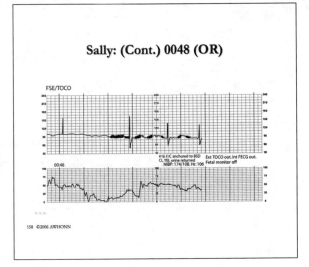

Sally: Outcome

■ Primary cesarean section with general anesthesia at 0103

■ Female infant; 4 lbs. 11 oz. (2126 gms)

■ Apgars 0/0/1/3

■ Full resuscitation x 11 minutes

■ Baby to NICU

■ Had one mild seizure in NICU

Sally: Outcome (Cont.)

Arterial blood gas results:

- pH   6.55   *mil acidotic*
- pO_2 11.4 mmHg
- pCO_2 127.8 mmHg   *60*
- HCO_3 10.6 mmHg
- BD: 32 mmol/L   *12 metabolic*

160 ©2006 AWHONN

Sally: Outcome (Cont.)
Couvelaire Uterus

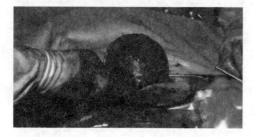

161 ©2006 AWHONN

Sally: Outcome (Cont.)

- Sally discharged home on day 4
- Infant discharged home on day 19
  - No apparent deficits
  - At 1 year of age, no neurological deficits noted

162 ©2006 AWHONN

Abruptio Placentae

- Pathophysiology
  - Premature separation of placenta
  - Associated with hypertension, preeclampsia
- Potential effects on fetus and mother
  - Uteroplacental insufficiency; loss of O_2 supply
  - Change in baseline FHR; decelerations or bradycardia
  - Increased uterine irritability and tonus
  - Bleeding, hemorrhage, shock

163 ©2006 AWHONN

Nadine, 15 years old
$G_1 P_0$, 36 $^2/_7$ weeks gestation

- Family History
  - Parents and maternal grandparents alive and well
  - No siblings
- Medical History
  - History of asthma last 2 years
  - Heart murmur
  - Chronic hematuria

164 ©2006 AWHONN

Nadine: Current Pregnancy

Current Pregnancy
- C/O dizziness for past two days
- C/O "wet panties"
- Labs: All within normal limits;
             ABO/Rh = A negative
- Hgb: 13.3 g/dL
- HbsAG, HIV, chlamydia, GC all neg
- + Group B strep at 32 weeks by urine culture

165 ©2006 AWHONN

Nadine: (Cont.) Admission Data

- Fern test confirmed SROM
- No uterine activity; no bleeding
- Fetal movement normal
- VS: BP 145/81, P 78, R 18, T 99.2° F (37.2 ° C)
- SVE: 2 cm/50%/-2
- Penicillin G 5 million units by IV piggyback
- Oxytocin started at 3 milliunits/min

166 ©2006 AWHONN

Nadine: Admission Tracing

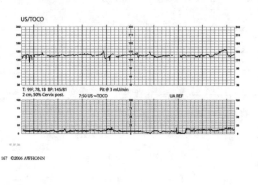

167 ©2006 AWHONN

Nadine: (Cont.) 1316

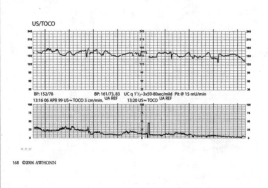

168 ©2006 AWHONN

Nadine: (Cont.) 1900

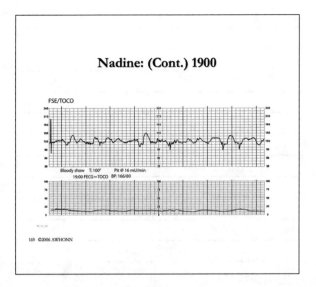

Nadine: (Cont) 1910

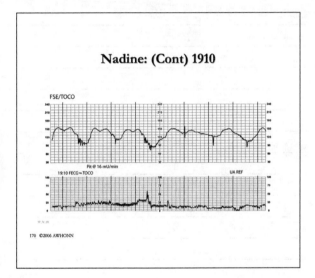

Nadine: (Cont) 2000

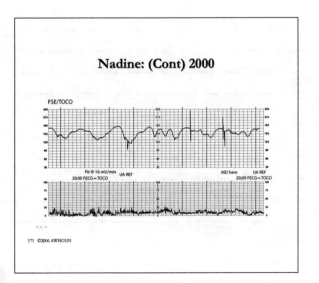

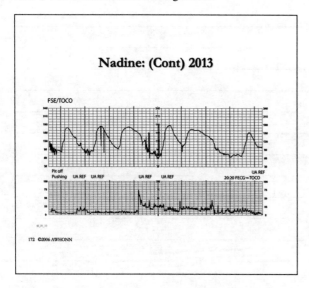

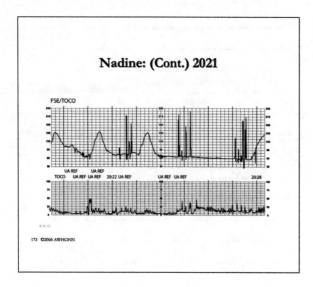

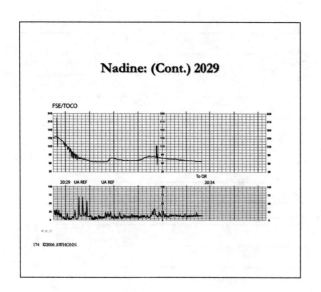

Nadine: (Cont.) In OR

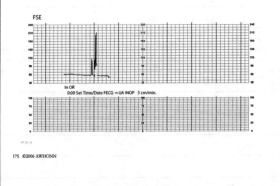

175 ©2006 AWHONN

Nadine: Outcome

- Cesarean birth at 2031
- Female infant; 7 lbs. 4 oz. (3288.5 gms)
- Apgars 1/1/intubated
- Enlarging cephalohematoma noted
- Full code x 20 minutes; pronounced in OR
- Uterus ruptured

176 ©2006 AWHONN

Uterine Rupture

Etiology
- Previous uterine scar
- Fetal, uterine anomalies
- Hx of placenta increta, percreta
- Mid-forceps delivery
- Fetal malpresentation
- Uterine hyperstimulation

Maternal-Fetal Effects
- Partial or complete uterine rupture
- Utero-placental insufficiency
- Fetal intolerance to labor
- Maternal hemorrhage
- Fetal injury, death

177 ©2006 AWHONN

Ginny, 30 years old
G3 P$_{1011}$ 37^5/$_7$ weeks' gestation

- Family History
  - Mother Type 2 diabetes
  - Father bladder cancer
- Medical History
  - History of human papilloma virus (HPV)
  - Latex allergy

178 ©2006 AWHONN

Ginny: History (Cont.)

- Previous Pregnancies:
  - Miscarriage 1991
  - Preeclampsia, postpartum hemorrhage
- Current Pregnancy:
  - Sudden onset of gross hematuria, nausea
  - Hospitalized for renal evaluation
  - Hydronephrotic kidney identified
  - Stent placed and morphine PCA initiated

179 ©2006 AWHONN

Ginny: Admission Data

Laboratory Tests
- WBC :   10.0 x 109/L
- Hct: 36%
- Platelets: 312K mm^3

180 ©2006 AWHONN

Ginny: Admission Data (Cont.)

- Vital signs:
  - ➤ BP 129/80, P 100, R 18, T 99°F, 37.2°C
- Cervix closed, thick; high station; vertex
- Contractions:
  - ➤ Q 3-4 mins; duration 60 seconds; moderate, soft resting tone
- FHR: Baseline 150 bpm; minimal variability

181 ©2006 AWHONN

Ginny: Admission Tracing

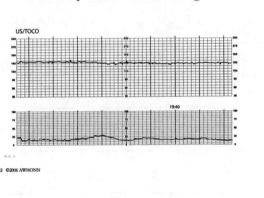

182 ©2006 AWHONN

Ginny: (Cont.) 0228

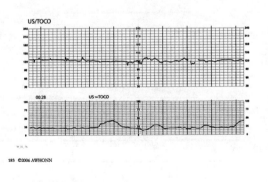

183 ©2006 AWHONN

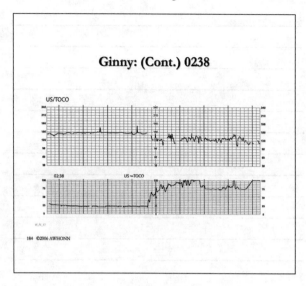

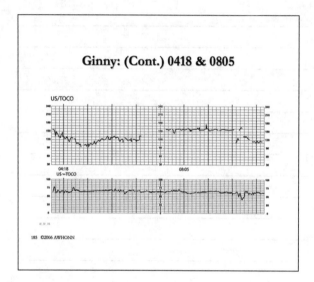

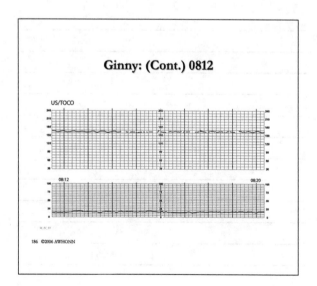

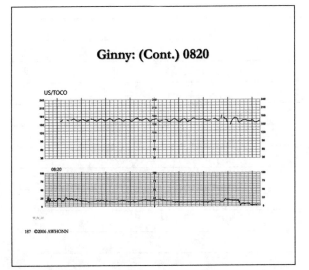

Ginny: (Cont.) 0820

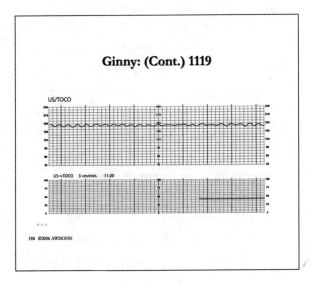

Ginny: (Cont.) 1119

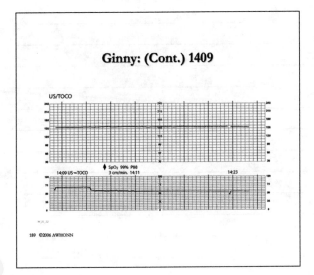

Ginny: (Cont.) 1409

Ginny: (Cont.) 1500

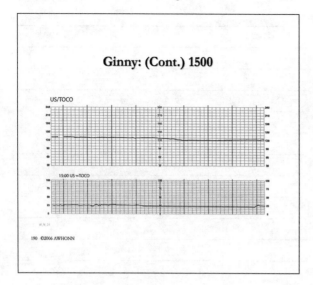

Ginny: (Cont.) 1540

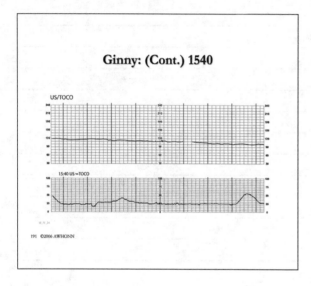

Ginny: Outcome

- Cesarean birth at 1559, under general anesthesia
- Male infant; 7 lbs., 14 oz. (3571 gms)
- Neonatal laboratory values:
  - Hematocrit: 19%   52-58%
  - Hemoglobin: 6.3 gm/dL   13-20
  - Red blood cells: $1.77 \times 10^{12}/L$
- Apgars: 1/1/1/2/4/5/7

Ginny: Outcome (Cont.)

- Arterial umbilical cord gas:
  - pH   6.77 ↓
  - pCO_2 58.0 ⊕
  - pO_2 19.0 ↓
  - HCO_3 9.0 ↓
  - BD   32 ↑
- Transfused 15 mL O negative blood

193 ©2006 AWHONN

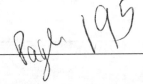

Page 195

Sinusoidal Patterns

- Pathophysiology:
  - Loss of oxygen supply
  - Loss of blood supply
- Resulting effects:
  - Fetal anemia
  - Potential for fetal compromise

194 ©2006 AWHONN

Summary

- Evaluate your patient's individual needs
- Assess all available information
- Communicate pertinent information
- Evaluate the effect of your actions

195 ©2006 AWHONN

**Documentation,
Communication
and Risk Management**

©2006 AWHONN

What Do You See?

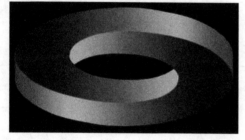

197 ©2006 AWHONN

What Is It?

- Standard
- Standards of nursing practice
- Standards of care
- Standards of professional performance

198 ©2006 AWHONN

Relationship to Nursing Process

- Standard
- Standards of nursing practice
- Standards of care
- Standards of professional performance

All relate to the nursing process (problem identification and solving process)

199 ©2006 AWHONN

Differentiating Standards from Guidelines

A guideline is a "framework developed through experts' consensus and review of the literature which guides patient-focused activities that affect the provision of care"

(AWHONN, 2003, p. 10)

- Standard = Principle of care provision
- Guideline = Suggested method of practice

200 ©2006 AWHONN

Examples of Sources of Standards

- AWHONN
- American College of Nurse Midwives (ACNM)
- ACOG
- SOGC
- AAP
- JCAHO
- Medicare and Medicaid

- American Nurses Association (ANA)
- National Association of Neonatal Nurses (NANN)
- Association of Operating Room Nurses (AORN)
- Royal College of Obstetrics and Gynecology (RCOG)

201 ©2006 AWHONN

Elements of Malpractice

- Duty
- Breach of duty
- Causation
- Damages
- Intervening cause or defense

202 ©2006 AWHONN

FHR Documentation
Based on Assessment Method

	Auscultation	External U/S	FSE
FHR	Rate Rhythm	Rate	Rate
Variability	N/A	Absent Minimal Moderate Marked	Absent Minimal Moderate Marked
Changes in FHR	Increases and decreases • Abrupt • Gradual	Accelerations Decelerations	Accelerations Decelerations

203 ©2006 AWHONN   (Adapted from Simpson & Knox, 2003)

Interventions Based on Physiologic Goals

	Max. placental blood flow	Max. umbilical circulation	Max. available oxygen	Reduce UA
Pos. change	v (lateral)	v	v (lateral)	v (lateral)
IV fluids	v			v
Medication	v (ephedrine or tocolytic)	v (consider tocolytic)		v (tocolytic)
↑ presenting part		v		
Amnio-infusion		v		
Maternal O2	v	v (if atypical)	v	
↓ uterotonics	v	v		v
Reduce pain & anxiety	v	v	v	v
Correct mat disease			v	
Guide breathing	v		v	v

204 ©2006 AWHONN

Sample Summary Narrative for Persistent Prolonged Deceleration

Excerpt of summary narrative:

"FHR BL 150 with moderate variability at 1315. Epidural in place at 1325. Prolonged FHR deceleration noted. Pt. position changed to L side, IV bolus 500 mL LR given, O2 at 10 L/min by non-rebreather mask on, MD notified. BP 90/60, pulse 92, RR 14. Ephedrine given per protocol. At 1338 no improvement in FHR baseline despite interventions. MD present. OR team notified to stand by for delivery…"

205 ©2006 AWHONN

Interventions for Prolonged Decelerations

- Alternate position changes
- Discontinue oxytocin or other uterotonic drugs
- Vaginal exam
- Elevation of presenting part
- Support for the mother, explain circumstances assist with breathing techniques
- Continue communication with primary care provider

206 ©2006 AWHONN

Definitions

- Assessment- the act of judgment of a person or a situation
- Documentation - writing that provides information, especially information of an official nature
- Evaluate - to measure or assess

207 ©2006 AWHONN

Suggested Assessment During Labor and Delivery

	First Stage	Second Stage
Maternal V S	At least q 4 hrs. (↑ PRN)	At least q 4 hrs. (↑ PRN)
FHR	Low risk q 30 min. / High risk q15 min.	Low risk q15 min. / High risk q 5 min.
	If EFM is continuously recording, periodic documentation may be used to summarize fetal status – per institution policy	

208 ©2006 AWHONN

Suggested Frequency for Auscultation

	Latent Phase	Active Phase	Second Stage
AWHONN		Q 15-30 min	Q 5-15 min
ACOG		Q 15 min	Q 5 min
RCOG		Q 15 min	Q 5 min
SOGC	Regularly after ROM or other clinically significant change	Q 15-30 min	Q 15 min, then Q 5 min once pushing initiated

(ACOG, 2005; AWHONN, 2005; Feinstein, Sprague and Trepanier, 2000; RCOG, 2001; SOGC, 2002)
209 ©2006 AWHONN

Suggested FHR Assessments with Procedures and Events

- Spontaneous or artificial ROM
- Allowing patient to ambulate
- Administration of medications such as antihypertensives, tocolytics
- Administration of analgesia or anesthesia
- Cervical exams
- Patient's return from ambulating or bathroom
- Recognition of abnormal patterns of uterine activity
- Administration of medications

(King-Urbanski & Cady, 1999)

210 ©2006 AWHONN

Suggested FHR Assessments with . . .

- Evaluation of analgesia or anesthesia
- Evaluation of oxytocin

(King-Urbanski & Cady, 1999)

211 ©2006 AWHONN

Considerations for Uterine Activity Assessment

Condition	Components and Assessment Frequency
No increased risk for complications	Frequency, duration, intensity, relaxation
While receiving augmentation	Frequency, duration, intensity, relaxation Before every dose increase, at least q hour if dose stable
While receiving Misoprostol	Frequency, duration, intensity, relaxation via continuous uterine monitoring
While receiving Cervidil	Frequency, duration, intensity, relaxation via continuous monitoring while in place and at least 15 min. after removed
While receiving Prepidil	Frequency, duration, intensity, relaxation via continuous uterine monitoring for at least 30 min. to 2 hours after placement

212 ©2006 AWHONN

Late Entries in the Medical Record

- Why?

- When?

- How?

213 ©2006 AWHONN

Late Entry Example

0930: Late entry for 0845.

Bradycardia to 80 bpm for 11 min. following epidural placement and dosing. Patient turned to left side, O2 applied at 10 L/min by non-rebreather mask, and IV bolus 500 ml LR and ephedrine given for BP of 90/52. Dr. Jones notified by phone of all changes in maternal/fetal status. FHR ↑ to BL of 140 bpm at 0857, with minimal variability for 25 min. At 0930 FHR baseline remains 140, now with moderate variability and no decelerations. Patient remains in side-lying position with O2 in place. Late entry due to need for emergent care.

214 ©2006 AWHONN

Documentation of Emergent Events

- Time FHR or maternal status recognized as nonreassuring
- Actions initiated for maternal or fetal resuscitation
- Continued assessment of fetal response to interventions
- Communication with team members and responses
- Time patient taken to the surgical suite and time of incision
- Chronologies of intervention performed (including by which personnel) for newborn resuscitation, if needed
- Narrative note reflecting discussion between health care providers and patient/family

215 ©2006 AWHONN   (Simpson & Knox, 2003)

Summary Documentation

1035: Summary late entry for 0910-0935.

SROM at 0910. Prolonged deceleration to 70 bpm. VE - prolapsed cord noted. Presenting part elevated, patient in knee-chest position. Emergency light activated. S. Smith RN & J. Jones RN to bedside. IV LR 700 ml bolus given, Dr. White called STAT to L&D, OR team notified. Anesthesia paged to OR STAT. Foley catheter placed. Bicitra 30 ml PO given. Dr. White in labor room, counseled patient & spouse about need for C/S birth en route to OR. Patient verbally consents to procedure. Patient in surgical suite at 0927, transferred to OR table. Presenting part kept elevated. FHR auscultated in OR at 105 bpm. Prep done. Anesthesia present & general anesthesia started. Incision time: 0935. See operative record & newborn assessment form for continued documentation.

216 ©2006 AWHONN

Documentation Challenges

- Double documentation
- Time synchronization

217 ©2006 AWHONN

Minimizing Liability Risk

Continuing education:

- Joint responsibility between nurses and employers
- Needed to:
  - Maintain competency in areas of practice
  - Obtain new knowledge
  - Incorporate new technology and skills into practice
  - Maintain awareness of current research as it applies to practice

(Simpson & Flood-Chez, 2001)

218 ©2006 AWHONN

Sources of Liability Claims

Cited Sources of Fetal and Neonatal Injury	Clinical Example
Failure to recognize and/or respond to antepartum and intrapartum fetal compromise	Misinterpreting EFM tracings
Delayed cesarean delivery (> 30 minutes from decision to incision) – for maternal-fetal indications	Communication difficulties between practitioners
Inability to appropriately resuscitate depressed infant	Supplies not readily available in rooms
Inappropriate use of oxytocin, misoprostol leading to uterine hyperstimulation, uterine rupture, fetal distress, fetal death	Laboring a woman attempting a VBAC
Inappropriate use of forceps/vacuum/fundal pressure leading to fetal trauma and/or preventable shoulder dystocia	Shoulder dystocia mis-managment

(Adapted from Simpson & Knox, 2003)

219 ©2006 AWHONN

JCAHO 2004 Recommendations

- Development of clear guidelines for fetal monitoring of potential high-risk patients, including nursing protocols for interpretation of fetal heart rate tracings

- Education of nurses, residents, nurse midwives, physicians to use standardized terminology to communicate abnormal fetal heart rate tracings

- Review of organizational policies regarding availability of key personnel for emergency interventions

220 ©2006 AWHONN

Additional Suggestions for Minimizing Liability Risk

- Document care provided

- Use medical record audit tools

- Practice according to guidelines

- Participate in and promote multidisciplinary quality management and policy development in your facility

(Simpson & Knox, 2003)

221 ©2006 AWHONN

Green/Yellow/Red: Risk Management

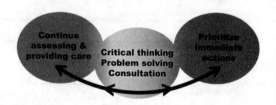

222 ©2006 AWHONN

Effective Communication

- Speaking clearly
- Being courteous and professional
- Presenting facts in a methodical or chronological format
- Asking for clarification if others' communication or orders are not clear
- Communicating recommendations for care

Effective Communication (Cont.)

- Communicate all relevant facts, abnormal findings and specific areas of concern.
- State reasons when there's a disagreement about the plan of care.
- If the mother and/or fetus are in danger, tell the care provider to report to the hospital immediately to assess the situation → document.
- Inform the provider if the chain of command is to be initiated.

(Sullivan & Bowden, 1999)

Chain of Command

- Patient care policies and procedures should be in place and accessible to nurses and physicians.

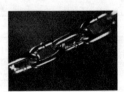

- Nurses and physicians should understand and know how to implement their facility's chain of command.

(Connors, 2003)

Sample Chain-of-Command

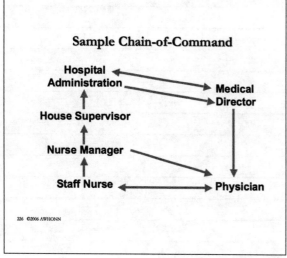

226 ©2006 AWHONN

JCAHO Sentinel Event Alert #30

Primary factors contributing to perinatal morbidity and mortality:

- Communication issues
- Organizational culture

(JCAHO, 2004)

227 ©2006 AWHONN

Julie: 26 years old
$G_3 P_{0112}$

- Family history:
  - Both parents, husband healthy
  - Twin sister died in childbirth, amniotic fluid embolus
- Medical/surgical history:
  - Latex allergy
- Previous pregnancy history:
  - Delivered twins vaginally at 36 weeks
  - Both boys healthy, age $3^1/_2$
- Psychosocial history:
  - Unremarkable

228 ©2006 AWHONN

Julie: Current Pregnancy

Antepartum

- Normal prenatal course
- HIV negative; group beta strep positive; A+; rubella immune; RPR neg.

Julie: (Cont.) Admission Data

- SROM 0800
- Admitted 1120
- FSE immediately applied after questionable auscultation of FHR at 90 bpm
- Cervix 4-5/90%/-1
- Contractions every 10-15 minutes, mild

Julie: (Cont.) 1130

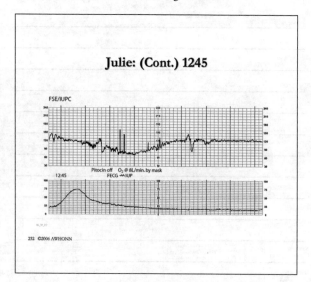

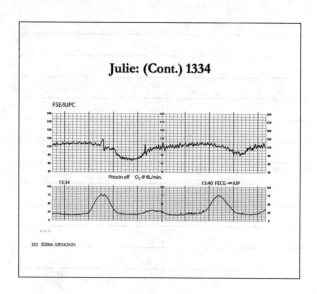

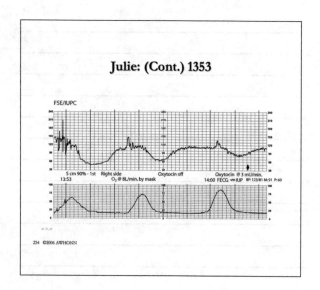

Discussion Items

- Documentation of conversation
- Is it reasonable to restart oxytocin?
- Nurse's liability: is it changed with MD present?
- What can the nurse do if still uncomfortable with the situation?

235 ©2006 AWHONN

Julie: (Cont.) 1420

FSE/IUPC

Oxytocin @ 5 mU/min.
14:20 FECG ➳IUP

236 ©2006 AWHONN

Julie: (Cont.) 1435

FSE/IUPC

Pushing @ 0 station   14:40 FECG ➳IUP

237 ©2006 AWHONN

Julie: (Cont.) 1450

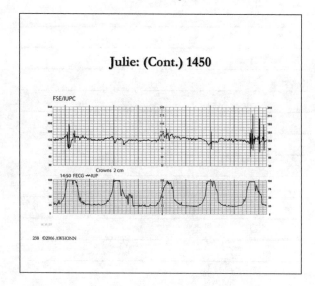

Julie: Outcome

- Spontaneous vaginal delivery
- No lacerations, no episiotomy
- Female 7 lbs., 2 oz. (3282 grams)
- Apgars 8/9/9

Discussion

Review of potential actions by the nurse:
- Refuse to continue oxytocin.
- Continue with chain of command.
- Documentation/communication.

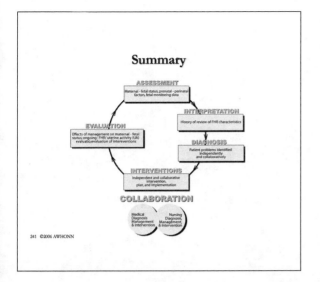

Summary

ASSESSMENT
Maternal - fetal status, prenatal - perinatal factors, fetal monitoring data

INTERPRETATION
History of review of FHR characteristics

EVALUATION
Effects of management on maternal - fetal status; ongoing- FHR/ uterine activity (UA) evaluation;evaluation of interventions

DIAGNOSIS
Patient problems identified independently and collaboratively

INTERVENTIONS
Independent and collaborative intervention, plan, and implementation

COLLABORATION

Medical Diagnosis Management & Intervention

Nursing Diagnosis Management & Intervention

241 ©2006 AWHONN